Advance Praise

Dr. Yani has done a fantastic job of giving her readers a solution to the ever increasing problem of stress, fatigue and decreased energy in a straight forward, easy to understand and easily implementable plan. She has taken 30 plus years of experience helping thousands of people regain their "life" and presented that gift to you in this guide to more energy, a healthier life and greater happiness! Begin your new life today!

~Dr Gary Fieber - CEO Maximum Performance
Solutions, 30 years chiropractic and acupuncture,
International lecturer and educator and
Consultant to Healthcare Providers

This book is smart and unique and written for the person who needs to overcome their fatigue and create a life that is great, filled with boundless energy and productivity.

~Roberta Swanson, CPA

This book is a gem!!! It's necessary and perfect for all levels of people no matter where they are at in their health. Dr. Yani's guidance is authentic, truthful, and very direct. She teaches you the eight steps to health, wellness and vitality in a very easy and useable way. I actually started while I was still reading the book! Thank you so much Dr. Yani for sharing your wisdom!

~Ammie Bowman, HHP

This is a must read for everyone wanting to improve their health and feel more energized. It was an easy read, for a non-medical background person as myself, very straight forward explaining from the cellular level, and most importantly it is do-able!!!!!

~Laura Verdugo, CARE Specialist Rio Hondo College

An extremely well-written guide to positively impact both men and women in all walks of life! This wonderful book outlines basic, yet fundamental building blocks that affect the whole person; mind, body and spirit. The book explains complex concepts in layman's terms, and is not over-complicated, which makes it a great read! A thoroughly enjoyable read that provides steps that anyone can take to improve their life-style and thrive, not just survive. Where has this book been all my life?

~Linda Aguirre, Legal Support Administrator for Dentons Los Angeles

Excellent book! It was so simple, short and clear!!! Thank you so much. I really appreciate your time and how much you sincerely care. Can't wait for the hard copy!

~Elizabeth Corona, Realtor

Your book is very educational and easy to read. I find it's full of practical advice without recommending a lot of complicated practices that might overwhelm and discourage a reader who really wants to make a serious attempt at getting better. I think you covered all the basis.

~Judy Daddieco

Dr. Yani's book, No More Fatigue, *offers a straightforward guide to improving one's energy and overall health. It is easy to read and chock full of many helpful gems and advice you can implement right away. The author presents her advice in easy to understand terms and examples that anyone can follow. I definitely recommend this book if you are looking for ways to improve your energy level and attain overall better health.*

~Sheilla Borromeo, Registered Nurse

No More Fatigue

NO
MORE
FATIGUE

The Guide to Increase Energy and Productivity in Everything You Do

DR. YANI FELICIANO

FOREWORD BY DICK WALKER, M.D., F.A.C.P., F.A.C.E.P.

NEW YORK

LONDON • NASHVILLE • MELBOURNE • VANCOUVER

No More Fatigue

The Guide to Increased Energy and Productivity in Everything You Do

Published in New York, New York, by Morgan James Publishing in partnership with Difference Press. Morgan James is a trademark of Morgan James, LLC. www.MorganJamesPublishing.com

ISBN 9781642797367 paperback
ISBN 9781642797374 eBook
ISBN 9781642797381 audio book
Library of Congress Control Number: 2019947239

Cover & Interior Design by:
Christopher Kirk
www.GFSstudio.com

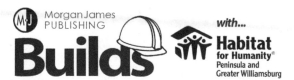

Morgan James is a proud partner of Habitat for Humanity Peninsula and Greater Williamsburg. Partners in building since 2006.

Get involved today! Visit
MorganJamesPublishing.com/giving-back

For Soren!

*Thank you for always encouraging me to live the life
I love helping my clients live the lives they love.*

Table of Contents

Foreword xiii
Introduction xix

Chapter 1   Fatigue Is a Modern Epidemic 1
Chapter 2   My Story 7
Chapter 3   Framework of Energy Steps 17
Chapter 4   Eating for Energy 21
Chapter 5   What's so Important About Water? 43
Chapter 6   Nutritional Supplements That Matter . . . 49
Chapter 7   Good Night and Sleep Tight 71
Chapter 8   Got Stress? 81
Chapter 9   Attitude, Feelings, and Law of
             Resonance 99
Chapter 10   How Does Exercise Increase Your
             Energy Levels? 109
Chapter 11   Plan Your Life and Manage Your Time . . 119

Chapter 12   Obstacles in Your Way 127
Chapter 13   Conclusion 133

Acknowledgements 137
Thank You 143
About the Author 145

Foreword

It is no secret that fatigue is a modern epidemic that affects so many people on this planet in profound ways. Yet nearly every day I hear stories of transformation that strengthen my faith that people can make simple changes and dramatically improve their health and wellbeing. I am a double board certified Internist and Emergency physician of 40 years and spent most of my career in the emergency room. I also have a master's degree in Preventive Medicine. This gives me a unique perspective in not only helping those patients that end up in the emergency room but more importantly how they can prevent many of the ailments that cause them to end up there. Unfortunately, as a medical doctor in the ER I do not have the time to help patients build healthy habits and help them implement what they need to do. I have to treat them as quickly and efficiently as possible because there are many others waiting to be seen. I have always considered myself an athlete and I have enjoyed having the energy to hike, ski and climb mountains, one of which was Mt. Everest. For the last 7 years, in addition to working in the ER, I have been encouraging people to take charge of their lives by improving their health. That's how I met Dr. Yani. I initially met her when a mutual friend, who is a holistic health practitioner, introduced us. I immediately thought to myself, "what a delightful person". I have gotten to know her better and have developed a friendship with her and her husband. She and I work closely with other doctors to assist them in helping more people who are struggling to overcome challenges and increase their energy and vitality. I can tell you that Dr. Yani cares deeply for her patients and clients she coaches. She is always finding ways to help those struggling with health challenges to change their lives for the better.

This book is full of practical information and action steps that the reader can take to enhance their energy and productivity in everything they do. Dr. Yani has been helping her patients and clients overcome their fatigue for over 30 years and has found safe and natural ways to help them accomplish this without putting them at risk. She is a doctor of chiropractic who can help her clients physically and give them recommendations but she goes even further by not only treating them in most cases but by helping them implement healthy lifestyle changes that they invariably needed to make sure that the correction sticks. She has been coaching her patients in what they need to do so they actually achieve the results they want. I have been to Dr. Yani's offices and have had the opportunity to interact with her patients and clients and I can tell you that they love her and trust her because she puts their needs first and foremost. She has a unique approach to helping people. She first helps them determine what they want to Be, Do and Have in their lives; then she designs an individual plan so they can achieve it by overcoming their challenges. That's the key to getting the best results. I've never seen anything like this before but the extra support she gives them is what is making a difference in their lives. I can see the pleasure in Dr. Yani's face when she talks about being able to make such a huge difference in her clients' lives. Dr. Yani wanted to write this book so that she could make an even greater impact on the world by making the information in the book available to more than those people she interacts with one on one. She details her story and then goes right into the 8 steps that are required in order to eliminate fatigue and increase productivity. The steps include eating high quality foods in the correct proportions and drinking enough water, at the right times, to stay abundantly hydrated. She outlines how important it is to not only give your body the building blocks it needs but the labor to get the job done. I love how she explains the need for rest and sleep as well as some stress reduction techniques that include the movement and stretching we need to do to correct injuries from postural imbalances. She even goes into productivity techniques, mindset, and the law of vibration, a universal law of which people are becoming more aware. She gives the reader choices on how they can accomplish health through cellular regeneration and gives examples of how increasing mitochondrial numbers and size can increase energy at a cellular level. In today's world we are doing more than we ever did before and have less time to get it all done. I believe the reader will definitely be able to change their unique circumstances to take their life to the next level. As she puts it, her ideal clients want to thrive not just survive.

My hope for you, the reader, would be for you to not only learn these valuable steps but take the action necessary to implement them in your life so that you too can build the momentum you need to transform your life. I can tell you that you may encounter obstacles that will derail your efforts to implement these simple steps, but I encourage you to persevere and know that you can do this. I am happy to speak from my heart and let you know you're in for a treat with this book. Good luck to you in following the advice on what to do and if you feel you need more support in doing the right things, I recommend you reach out to Dr. Yani. She works with clients to make the necessary shifts from unhealthy habits to healthy habits. She helps her patients and clients not only follow her recommendations but she tailors the recommendations to their individual situation which yields the greatest results. Dr. Yani has helped thousands of people get the results they wanted in life and she can help you too.

Dick Walker, M.D., F.A.C.P., F.A.C.E.P.
DickWalkerMD.com

Introduction

I wrote this book because I saw too many people suffering with severe issues that zapped their energy and vitality, and I saw that they were hurting physically and in other aspects of their lives. When you suffer physically, you will also suffer mentally and in your marriage and at work, basically in your whole life. I saw how their poor health was ruining their lives and the lives of their children. They just couldn't see it or didn't know what to do about it.

I was sad to see the suffering of others. As a doctor, I naturally wanted to help improve their lives. I wanted to bring joy and happiness to the millions of people who were suffering. I was, in fact, doing that in my own chiropractic practice on a smaller scale, but I wanted to reach more people with my message of love and healing, more people than I could see in the practice one-on-one.

I am undeniably driven to help people. It is my calling. When I'm helping people, I feel alive. I want you to feel alive, too. I know there are people out there in the world that are still having challenges and I want to offer them the help I have offered to thousands in my 30+ year career in private practice. Before I was able to help them, most of my patients complained of energy issues, particularly when they have pain or sleep issues and stress. I knew I could help them and I know I can help you. I want to share those ideas with you so that you, too, can benefit.

It made me sad to see Joanie's struggle in her life. I knew that I could help her if she trusted me and followed my recommendations. I knew I needed to help her take the action steps to be able to change her life. So many people want to be helped but they don't do what is needed to get the results they want. I promise you that I will do my best to teach you the exact steps that will help you really get better and be able to live the life you want. I want you to feel great and be super productive in everything you do. So I will be taking you by the hand and educating you on all the steps to do so. But more importantly, I want to encourage you to actually take the action you need to take.

I want to help you with all the reasons that are holding you back from achieving all your goals and dreams. First, however, you'll need to fix your fatigue. Fatigue is not a single condition, but a symptom that shows up due to a variety of issues. I can tell you that I have helped many people just like you gain greater energy and vitality. All you need to do is follow the instructions put forth in this book. Please keep an open mind, and follow your heart. Know that I have your best interests in mind and want what is best for you so that you can feel great and be super productive again.

I want you to learn what you need to do to overcome your fatigue and why you need to do it. But more importantly, I want you to take action. If you only gain the knowledge but you don't take the necessary action and apply the steps I will be sharing, then this book will not make a difference in your life. Trust the process and trust me because I have helped thousands of people just like you achieve their dreams of being happy and healthy and super productive. I want to help you make the necessary changes that you need to make so that you can have all your dreams come true. It is absolutely possible, and I will walk you through all the steps to make it happen. My mission in life is to help you improve your life.

I have helped others achieve great results with boosting energy and productivity through workshops, speaking engagements, and one-on-one sessions. I promise not to leave you hanging to figure out these concepts on your own, but to walk you through them so that you know exactly what to do. That way, you can incorporate them easily and understand the "why" behind them. I have found that when you know the why, then you comply. When you comply, then you get the results you want.

***

Fatigue is rampant in today's society. So many people suffer from a lack of energy and it doesn't have to do so much with age but with lifestyle. The good news is that you will understand exactly what is missing or needs to be tweaked in your life so that you can have an amazing breakthrough.

Some of the principles in this book seem simple, but you need to follow them nonetheless. Each step is very specific. Some things can be altered, but for the most part, you need to follow the steps as closely as written. I have applied these methods myself and with thousands of people, and I know that they produce amazing results.

In this book, I offer my advice on how you can feel great and be super productive in everything you do. If you are concerned about how any of these methods may affect your current health, you should consult your doctor before making any changes.

My goal is to help you live a happy and healthy life with greater energy and productivity. It's time to take your life to a higher level. Today is your day! You can do this.

Chapter 1

Fatigue Is a Modern Epidemic

"The higher your energy level, the more efficient your body. The more efficient your body, the better you feel, and the more you will use your talent to produce outstanding results."
– Anthony Robbins

Peak performers are bursting with energy. They set out to accomplish all their goals, and they succeed. When you have energy, you have vitality and you can set your mind to doing everything that needs to be done to move in a direction to achieve all your hopes and dreams. By keeping your energy levels high, you gain a head start on fulfilling your dreams. Energy leads you to thrive, not just survive. Unfortunately, so many people are suffering right now with a lack of energy, some with extreme exhaustion. They can't figure out what to do, and they see their hopes and dreams disappearing right in front of them. A lack of energy gets in the way of you fulfilling all your hopes and dreams. What kind of life can you really have if you're so tired that you can hardly meet the minimum requirements of your day?

You are not alone. Over 90 percent of people I have surveyed say they don't have the energy they would like to have. So many people need help with this. They need to know what to do before their lives are ruined. They need to decide that enough is enough. They need to make a change and do things differently than what they are doing now in order to produce a different outcome.

"I just don't have the energy I need to perform my job."

"I don't have the energy to work and then come home to take care of my husband."

"I'm struggling with a sense of needing to sleep all the time because I just don't have the energy to stay awake."

"I'm exhausted at the end of the day and just collapse on my couch every night when I get home."

These were the words Joanie told me when she came to see me. Joanie is a 52-year-old CPA that lives in Southern California. She used to enjoy hiking with her husband and Labrador named Maxine, "Max" for short. She has many corporate clients and for her, it was crunch time. She is brilliant with numbers. She is trying her best to do her job but her fatigue is out of control. She is struggling to get the job done. She has many clients and is super busy. She loves what she does, but sitting at a computer all day is killing her neck and back. She's exhausted all the time. She tries to eat well, but she finds herself eating fast foods, and she doesn't have the time or energy to work out like she used to. She's put on an extra 20 pounds. She would like to be healthy, but finds herself working all the time. At this point, even if she had the time, she wouldn't have the energy.

She is married to her high school sweetheart Bob, a commercial contractor who travels a lot. She does not have any kids. She confided in me that there is no way she could do anything more than what she's doing now. Joanie's biggest problem is that she is overwhelmingly fatigued, and she's afraid to lose her corporate accounts. On top of that, she has some aches and pains in her neck and shoulders that occur when she's at her desk. She has had issues with sciatica at times too. She related that she is mostly worried about her severe lack of energy and wanted to know if it was related to her hormones being out of whack, or maybe something else that was seriously wrong. She sometimes can't even get out of bed in the morning due to the pain and feeling of exhaustion.

What keeps her up at night is the pain and fatigue, which are distracting her from doing her job, and it seems like it is getting worse. She is seriously worried that she is not going to meet her deadlines and her clients won't get the accounting services they need and will look for someone else. Not solving this problem is ruining her life personally and professionally. She doesn't feel like doing anything, and she is worried her health is deteriorating due to her lack of healthy habits.

She used to enjoy her work, but now it's becoming a drag, and she has had to hire an assistant to help her keep up. If she doesn't get the help she needs, she will continue the downward spiral she's in, and quite frankly, she's scared that ultimately, she's going to find herself unable to balance her professional life and her personal life as her health further deteriorates. Joanie just can't take it anymore. With the risk of losing her job, Joanie asked me to help her get her fatigue under control.

Without my help, she would've continued to rely on medications for her pain and lots of coffee and other stimulants to help her make it through the day. She soon realized that they will not fix her problem. She cried when she was able to see, maybe for the first time, just how bleak her future looked without getting her fatigue under control. There was a glimmer of hope for her as she wiped the last tear from her cheek. It had been so long that she had almost forgotten what hope felt like. If only she could get her fatigue under control, she could then reach other life goals and dreams.

That's why Joanie needed me. She needed me to help her get her life back on track so that she could feel energy and vitality again and be able to feel great and be super productive at work. She needed me to show her what to do so that she could be happy again and really live her life to the fullest without any more regrets. Joanie was a strong person and, despite feeling so tired all the time, she refused to give up on herself. So I showed Joanie what I'm going to show you. I showed Joanie what it would take to be able to feel great and be super productive at work and be happy so she could have the life she truly wanted. A life she truly loved. And I'm going to show that to you, too, in the following pages

Chapter 2

My Story

I became passionate about health and wellness, helping people to improve their lives, when I was young. I was born with a heart murmur, a congenital interventricular septal defect, IVSD. It was a tiny hole between the ventricles of my heart. They said it was the size of a pin hole. The doctors said I should grow out of it when I became a teenager, but I never quite did. Being raised in the military with free medical services, my parents took me into the doctor whenever they said I should go. It was like clockwork. I had to have blood tests, echocardiograms, EKGs, and whatever they decided. I always dreaded it. As a child, I had no choice, but as I got older, they kept wanting to do more and more tests. It was always the same thing. The heart murmur was still there, blood work the same, etc. I felt like a normal kid, but they were always making such a big deal out of it.

My heart murmur wasn't going away, and when I became a teenager they recommended cardiac catheterization, which they explained to me as cutting an inch incision in my groin and sticking a tube in through there up to my heart to take pictures and check it out. I am a girl that had a problem with a simple blood test, there was no way I was going to allow that. I just flat out refused, and said I wasn't going back to see anyone again. I was done. I didn't understand why I had to keep having tests for them to write little notes in my chart and never do anything anyway. The whole medical system to me didn't feel right. Maybe they're good about helping you when you're sick, but I wasn't getting anything out of it other than being traumatized because they always wanted blood. I informed my mom that I would no longer be going to these medical appointments, and so I stopped. Something inside me wanted to be a doctor someday because maybe I thought I could be different and not torture people in the process (maybe subconsciously), but that wasn't going to happen because doctors had to cut people and poke them with needles. There was no way I could do that.

Fast forward to my freshman high school year. When I graduated, I didn't know what I wanted to be. I liked to travel, so when my choir teacher asked me what I wanted to be, I said "maybe I should be a flight attendant so I could travel the world." It's funny, but she poo pooed my idea and said that I was smart and I loved helping people and I should be a doctor. I immediately shut that idea down because I didn't want to work with needles or blood.

By the time I was in my last year of high school, I fell in love. I was almost 17. He was a Greek military police officer that I met on the base when I would go in and out of the gate. Half way through my senior year, my dad moved us from Louisiana to Virginia. I was not happy to say the least. I didn't know anyone, and coming to a new school four and a half months before I graduated sucked! I had enjoyed all the travel the military allowed me up until then. I had a long-distance relationship with my fiancé. I was beginning to wonder if that was my dad's plan all along. Long story short, it was the best thing that happened to me, but I wasn't going to realize that for a few years. I put my head down and went to school and got an education. I didn't have a passion for any one thing because I really didn't know what I wanted to do. My dad suggested I take general education classes and I'd find my passion later. While getting a general education, I continued my long-distance relationship. I met a judo player who was training for the 1984 Olympics who was in the army. He was a great guy and I told him my fiancé was on the military judo team too. It turns out they knew each other, and when he found out who my fiancé was, he was less than complimentary about him. Turns out, my fiancé had several girlfriends in different towns where they traveled to play judo. I was devastated.

That was it. I was done. I was heartbroken. I had no idea what I was going to do, but I knew one thing – I didn't want to ever depend on a man. The good news was that I stayed in school and I kept accumulating credits. While in school for clinical nutrition, I met Patti, a wonderful woman who would become my mentor. She was a chiropractor and lived a few doors down from my apartment on Newbury Street in Boston. She was amazing, and my sister and I met her at a whole life expo because we worked for a women's bodybuilding gym. She wanted to check our spines. I had been working out running and weightlifting, so I didn't think I had any problems. But I was curious, nonetheless. She did find a few things that were misaligned. Since I was totally into health and wellness, I felt that I should get it fixed. I loved her, and although I didn't feel I had any major problems, it was amazing how much better and more energized I felt after starting chiropractic care.

Patti was an amazing chiropractor. She was an independent woman who I looked up to. After receiving treatments form her for a while, she needed help in the front office part-time when her other employee couldn't make it. I jumped at the opportunity. I learned so much, and every time I went to her office either to be seen as a patient or work for her, I came alive. I absolutely fell in love with helping people. There was so much satisfaction in seeing people's lives change. Patti saw a change in me and trained me to prep the patients for her. I'd give them a mini massage before she was ready for them, and I loved it! People were commenting on my healing hands and they suggested I should be a chiropractor. Patti agreed. I knew I had found my calling and passion, so I immediately called my parents and told them the news. They were always supportive, and it was a turning point in finding my dream and getting over my heartbreak. It was like flipping a switch. I went from just attending school classes to being on fire. So getting my heart broken was actually the best thing that ever happened to me! I immediately began the process to enroll in chiropractic school, and luckily, due to my dad's guidance, I had all the general education credits I needed except anatomy and physiology, physics, and organic and inorganic chemistry, which I enrolled in while still in Boston. I have never looked back. I love seeing people happy, and there's nothing like making a difference in someone's life.

I didn't really feel like I had a severe fatigue issue myself, but I have helped many people with this issue. They don't always come to me with that as their main complaint, but it quickly becomes apparent that it is a real issue for them. Hardly anyone has just one thing wrong with them. It is often a blend of conditions which manifest in many different ways.

In my early twenties and into my thirties, I did have an issue that I didn't think was bad but it was kind of annoying. I always thought I was a morning person because I woke up with the sunrise and I could rarely stay up late like other people. It was something that all my friends were aware of and they dismissed it as being "me." I had a habit of falling asleep during or shortly after dinner. When at the dinner table, after I ate, I would get tired and sleepy. And if I didn't get up and go to bed or lay down on the couch or anything else, I'd fall asleep right then and there. It was no big deal to me because for the most part, it didn't matter. The stressful thing was that, if there was an outing or a dinner party or any occasion where I needed to stay awake, it was so hard. I would politely apologize and tell whoever I was with that I was a morning person and it was past my bedtime. It was embarrassing at times when I would give anything to lay down but I was at someone else's house and I couldn't. I had to plan my life around the clock because I knew that shortly after dinner I would turn back into a pumpkin.

If I wanted to go to the movies with friends then it had to be an early show because I would never be able to stay awake if it started after 8. Once I had gone skiing with my girlfriends to Jackson Hole Mountain Resort in Wyoming and we stopped at the Million Dollar Cowboy bar because we thought it was cool since the bar stools were western riding saddles. I think we were waiting to order some food and I was feeling a bit tired and I fell asleep with my head on the bar counter. My girlfriends were used to it so they didn't think anything about it and had fun and woke me up when they were ready to leave.

The people there thought I was drunk. But that was not the case. That was just my thing.

The good news is that I later learned it was related to how I was eating, and that rarely happens now. In fact, the energy I have now is amazing, and sometimes I have to remind myself to go to sleep because it's 1 or 2 a.m., and I know that I will be rising with the sun no matter what time I go to bed. More about that later.

When I was pregnant with my daughter, I would work every day until 7 pm and thank God I lived close because sometimes I would walk in the door and go straight to bed. I developed a routine to help me cope with that which allowed me to work until the day before I delivered my beautiful daughter. I had her on Friday morning and was back to work by Monday. This is not what I recommend for others, but in those days I was a workhorse and, because I loved my job, it didn't seem like work. The only drawback was that I missed that little girl. I just wanted to hold her in my arms all day long. Luckily, in the early days, I lived on the same block as my office. And my mother stayed with me the first month or so and would bring her up the block for her feeding. I breast fed for over a year. This was the first time in my career that I loved two things with all my heart, and they were on opposite ends of the spectrum. I loved going to work and helping people solve their health and wellness problems. I felt alive! And I loved spending time holding my baby girl and looking into her big brown eyes.

I had the absolute best of both worlds, and tried to manage my time to make it work. I worked long hours but spent time with my sweet baby also. Good thing I had my own practice and could make my own hours. However, as my business flourished, I felt guilty spending time away from my daughter, and though I did spend every minute of time I wasn't working with her, it never seemed to be enough. I tried to solve the problem initially by buying a house a few doors down from my office that I would later convert into a home office. The project took two years to complete, but it was amazing. I lived above and worked below and I was able to see my daughter while I worked. It was like a dream come true! I was so happy and so was my daughter. I was able to balance my personal and professional life for the most part.

For 3 years, all was going well, and then my first husband and I divorced. My daughter and I would be hanging out alone. Those were bonding years for us. Life for me was very rewarding because I was living the life I loved and I was spending time with my daughter. This went on for four years, until I woke up one day feeling like something was missing and I prayed to God and said I was ready to open my heart up again but please take care of me and my daughter and only put someone in my path that fits my description. And while I'd love to say I wanted someone tall, dark, and handsome, my greatest concern was that he be of high moral and ethical character. I was ready to open my heart, and that was when

I met my husband. Now I have everything that fills my heart with joy. Fast forward twenty years, and I live a wonderful life helping make a difference in others' lives while enjoying the company of my husband and visiting my daughter, her husband, and my three grandchildren as often as possible in Washington State.

Chapter 3

Framework of Energy Steps

Now that you know fatigue is a modern epidemic causing millions of people to suffer needlessly, I would like to share with you ways to increase your energy beyond what you can imagine by taking in consideration that there is a scientific way to blow your energy through the roof and it begins with our cells.

Too many people put up with their fatigue until they just can't take it anymore. Then they make a change which sometimes takes years. It's a choice you have to make. It is easy to make a change once you decide to, but it's also easy not to do anything and stay the same. The question is: where are you now, and where do you want to be? Take a close look and ask yourself, do I want to live a better life? Am I unhappy with my energy levels?

If you answered yes or absolutely, then you should decide to make a change.

This book is filled with action packed ways to make changes that are going to get you from where you are to where you want to be. I present eight different ways to increase your energy levels and productivity. These steps are not in any particular order, and you can pick and choose which steps you want to start with first, but you will have to follow all the steps eventually if you want to get the best results.

Step One: I explain exactly how to eat the right foods in the right proportions to enhance your energy levels and not get into the food coma that so many people struggle with after eating their foods in the wrong proportions. You will understand why eating the right foods in the right proportions at the right times is critical for feeling great and being super productive at work.

Step Two: I lay out everything you need to know about water intake and how it helps you gain the most amount of energy. You will understand how drinking the right amount of water and the right type of water, and knowing when water should be consumed is critical for feeling great and being super productive on or off the job.

Step Three: I discuss how supplements can help you have the most ideal levels of energy and vitality. You will understand whether you actually need to take vitamins, minerals, antioxidants, or redox signaling molecules to feel great and be super productive in everything you do.

Step Four: I go over the differences in sleep and rest, and what you should do to maximize both to increase your energy. You will understand the difference between resting and sleeping and the effect it will have on your energy, and what you need to do to truly feel great and be super productive in everything you do.

Step Five: I put forth strategies to decrease physical, mental, and neurological stress on the body and increase energy by explaining the different stress reduction therapies that are available and how they work. You will understand the effects of stress on the body physically as well as mentally, and how to minimize the effects as much as possible so that you can feel great and be super productive in everything you do.

Step Six: I focus on the mindset necessary to move into higher frequencies and be in resonance with what you want to accomplish. You will understand that managing your feelings plays an important role in helping you to feel great and be super productive on and off the job.

Step Seven: I discuss the importance of moving and breathing and how different action steps can move us closer to boosting our energy levels, accomplishing what we want. You will understand that exercise and stretching is imperative in helping you feel great and be super productive at work, and there are simple hacks you can do to fit it into your schedule.

Step Eight: I show simple methods to mastering time management so that you will eliminate most of your mental stress, and help you not only feel great, but be super productive in everything you do.

These eight steps are easy steps to learn, but you may experience some resistance to change because what you're doing currently is familiar and safe. Yet, if you can decide to make the necessary changes, you will allow yourself to experience the full rewards. You will be able to reap the rewards of having greater energy and vitality and being super productive in everything you do. Be ready, willing, and able to make a change. That will set you up for success. My wish for you is for you to get to the end of the book and know that you have all the tools you need to be successful on your own, but if you would like my help, please reach out to me.

It's time to get started learning the steps you'll need to improve your energy and productivity so that you can feel great and be super productive on and off the job.

Chapter 4

Eating for Energy

Eating the right foods in the right proportions at the right time is critical to feeling great and being super productive on and off the job. You can't eat a bunch of crap and expect to feel awesome. Your body is your temple, and you want to treat it right. It's the body you get to live in for the rest of your life. I like to have a formula when it comes to eating food. My formula is you should eat to live, not live to eat.

My husband believes food should taste great and he enjoys eating. He likes to eat out and experience all the great foods at all the different restaurants. When he finds good ones, that's all he can talk about while trying to get me to try all these different places, too. Funny how opposites attract, because I like food as much as the next person, but my belief is I have to eat something to keep me going and doing all the things I want to do. It's great if it tastes good, but I prefer it to be healthy than delicious and filled with the "poisons" I have on my do not eat list. Given what I have learned over the last thirty-two years in practice and in being a health and wellness consultant, I want to be as healthy as possible. I think more people should strive to be the same. Now, there's an exception to this rule on holidays and birthdays and if a loved one slaved over the hot stove to prepare a nice meal, but for the most part, eating healthy is what I strive for. It's how I coach my patients and clients. Eat foods that aren't altered in any way. If it comes out of the ground or off a tree or roams around (I'm not a vegetarian yet, although I think I could be someday), then I'm good with that. The bottom line is I want to eat foods as close as possible to their natural form, not after being processed so much that you really can't tell what it was. I realize people want to eat bread and pasta and all these different types of processed foods. You can, at times, sure. But I recommend natural, whole foods that either don't have a huge list of ingredients or they have very few items on that list. I have found that foods that are over processed zap the energy out of you and cause issues due to all the chemicals, pesticides, herbicides, additives, and preservatives, etc. There are more toxic chemicals now than ever, and it is polluting our world and our bodies and our minds. More on that later.

Ask Yourself, How Processed Is This?

Eat foods that don't have labels, and if they do, read the labels. We live in a time when we are stressed out and don't have time to cook nice meals. I get that you're on the road and don't have a lot of time to prepare good food the way you might want to, but I don't think you should live off fast food and deli meat, for instance, that have a bunch of ingredients and are injected with mass quantities of sodium and sugar. In a pinch, we all might have to eat that way from time to time. What I'm saying is don't make these your go-to meals.

Plan Your Meals

We have to plan our meals if we want to be healthy and have them available to us so that we don't get stuck and have to eat the junk. I personally would rather skip a meal than go through a fast food drive-through. Although I must say, I've been told they are now including healthier choices than before. When I have my meals planned in advance, I don't have to skip anything. I have my husband make me chicken breast on the barbeque since I don't cook. And all he uses to marinate it is lemon, maybe a pinch of pepper. I personally don't like all those sauces, spices, marinades, etc. And funny thing is, I can always tell when he puts anything else on there. At first, he used to like to make it his way and try to secretly add marinades, but I could always tell the difference. And quite frankly, I just don't want anything added on my meat. I don't want preservatives and other stuff on my food. I find it amazing how tasty food really is when you can actually taste the food and it is not smothered in sauces, etc. You get the picture. You must start with healthy foods.

Macronutrients

Most foods fall into one of three categories: proteins, carbohydrates, and fats. We call them macronutrients. Proteins are amino acids that are building blocks for every cell, tissue, and organ in our body. They are foods like meat, poultry, seafood, eggs, milk (also carbohydrate), nuts (also fats), seeds, beans, and some vegetables, like peas. They actually provide the structure and support for our 70 plus trillion cells, so they are vital to our health! If you're not getting enough protein to help build your body, then your body will break down its own muscle tissue. Making up for that lack of protein causes a loss of energy and can cause weakness and pain in your muscles. So you need to think of proteins as being absolutely required for growth and repair of your body.

Carbohydrates are foods like bread, pasta, cereal, broccoli, potatoes, rice, fruits, and sweets, of course. When you eat carbohydrates, they are broken down into simple sugars that our body uses as fuel throughout the day. The best types of carbs to eat are the ones with lots of fiber in them, not the sugary treats you might prefer. Did you know that if you're having a problem with energy, then you're probably eating way too many carbohydrates as compared to proteins, and probably the wrong type? Eating too many carbs has been linked to diseases in the cardiovascular system, diabetes, and of course fatigue. However, when you eat carbohydrates in the proper proportion with proteins and fats, they could give you a ton of sustained energy and make you feel super healthy and productive.

The funny thing is, you unquestionably need to have fats and proteins in your diet in order to live. It's vital for your body to be able to function normally. That being said, some of you are really going to hate me for this, but you don't really need carbohydrates to live, especially not those of the sugary variety. You can survive just fine without them. Now I'm not going to tell you to eliminate all carbohydrates here, so relax. I believe that eating good quality carbohydrates, proteins, and fats in the proper proportion is essential for you to live with an abundant amount of energy, and that's what we'll be concentrating on in this book. And by the way, when I talk about not needing carbohydrates to survive, I'm talking about not needing bread, pasta and sugar. You don't need these types of carbohydrates as mentioned above. But I believe a healthy diet should have whole, natural, unprocessed foods such as vegetables and fruit in it… which are also carbohydrates!

Good Carbs

Think of making better choices and including whole-food, unprocessed carbs full of fiber like whole grains – quinoa, oats, brown rice, and buckwheat. Vegetables and fruits like sweet potatoes, potatoes (not French fries or potato chips), beets, squash, bananas, blueberries, apples, and oranges are super healthy. Nuts and seeds like almonds, walnuts, macadamia nuts, chia seeds, and pumpkin seeds are great. Legumes like cooked kidney beans, lentils, and garbanzo beans are beneficial, as well as broccoli and kale. Explore a variety of healthy, whole-food, unprocessed carbs.

Bad Carbs

Avoid processed and refined carbohydrates full of sugar like sugary beverages and fruit juices as well as pastries, cookies, and other baked goods. White bread, white rice, and white pasta should be avoided, and can be replaced with sprouted wheat bread, brown rice, and wheat pasta. Reduce or eliminate sugary treats like ice cream, candy, and mild chocolate, but remember that dark chocolate in moderation is good for you.

Fats

Fats are vital to us for many of our bodily functions. Fats give us energy, and we use it as fuel when we aren't burning sugar. Fats are essential to help us absorb certain vitamins which are essential to everyday life such as vitamin A (for healthy eyes and vision), Vitamin D (keeps bones strong by helping to absorb calcium), Vitamin E (protects your cells against free radical damage) and Vitamin K (helps with blood clotting).

Good fats help to protect your heart. Remember good fats help your heart and bad fats can increase heart disease. Ladies, fats help you produce the hormones you need and help with keeping your joints healthy, making them stay lubricated and move better, and slowing down the degenerative process over time. With all these benefits, thank God that fats are found pretty much in most of the foods you eat, to some degree. I'm sure you've heard that there are good fats and bad fats. I like to have as many clean fats as possible going into my body. Did I mention I love avocados? I can eat them as a snack. Just peel and eat. I'm getting hungry. If you put good fats in, then your body can release the bad fats that might be stored in your body and around your hips and thighs! Bad fats can cause all sorts of problems, including severe drain on your energy and problems with clogging your arteries, etc. Healthy fats are things like extra virgin olive oil (try to buy first cold pressed), chia seeds, avocados (yum, my favorite), dark chocolate, oily fish (like mackerel, tuna, and salmon), nuts, etc.

Fats are good for your brain! They keep your brain functioning so that you can think, and when eaten in the proper proportion, can help you manage your moods and help keep you energized. I always recommend you stay away from inflammatory types of fats and foods like anything fried (French fries), burgers, processed meats like hotdogs and sausages, and never eat margarine, shortening, or lard. These foods not only zap your energy, but increase inflammation in your body, which is bad for your heart, and they make your joints and body hurt. When you're in pain, that will zap your energy mentally and physically. When you eat clean and healthy fats in the correct proportion with carbohydrates and protein, they can increase your general energy and overall health and wellbeing. When you eat your foods in the proper proportions and they are healthy foods, you will find you're full of energy and vitality and you can get through the day with plenty of energy. You'll find that you are winning in life.

***

Unfortunately, that's not the case for everyone, and I have had patients who tell me that they almost had an accident on their way to work because they were daydreaming while driving. Have you ever left your house to go to work, and all of a sudden you were at work and couldn't even remember the trip? I can say this has happened to me at times. What happens is you mentally phase out of consciousness into not being fully aware of your surroundings, or you get into a trance-like state. This can be you at your desk daydreaming or, if you're in the car commuting, this could be a huge problem for you because it could be super dangerous if someone were to veer into your lane and you had to react quickly. If you're tired and not focused fully on the task at hand, it can have severe detrimental consequences. Your brain is fascinating, and I've heard that your subconscious brain can process millions of bits of information per second versus your conscious brain. Nevertheless, daydreaming while driving is dangerous and unacceptable.

The time that you spend less than fully conscious can be attributed to not eating your foods (proteins, carbs, and fats) in the proper proportion, or eating poor quality, highly processed foods. There's a reason for the daydreaming or what you might call a black out period or brain fog. When you eat a meal that's too high in carbohydrates, it causes your body to secrete insulin (and the reason your body secretes insulin is because it needs to bring down your blood sugar levels. That's a normal thing and it happens every time you eat too many refined carbs that spike your insulin. What would happen if your blood sugar levels continued to increase unchecked? You will die!). Insulin causes the blood sugar level to drop back down to the baseline. Your blood sugar and insulin levels don't drop down at the same time, so it actually causes this blackout period, or what you would consider brain fog, fatigue, etc. You get tired and can't think properly, your productivity lessens, and you feel like, "gosh, I've got to run and get some coffee and a donut or candy bar or something that will perk me back up." When you eat that snack, you're consuming more carbohydrates, which causes your blood sugar to increase again. It triggers another insulin spike, and they both (blood sugar and insulin levels) fall again at different speeds, producing a second episode of brain fog. Now it's lunch time, and maybe you go out with a friend and have some pasta for lunch. You even try to eat a salad before your pasta so you can feel healthy, and you order a soda or lemonade as a drink, and you couldn't pass up the yummy dessert, so you split it. Carbohydrates, carbohydrates, carbohydrates and more carbohydrates. A meal like this may give you a bit of energy initially, but think about it. Everything you just ate was primarily carbohydrates, with maybe a bit of fat in the salad dressing and in your dessert. By the time you get back to work, you will be in a food coma because of the blood sugar and insulin spike. Or maybe you go to a burger joint, and you decide you'd like to have a hamburger, Coke, and fries. The bread is a carbohydrate, the meat is a protein (yay), the fries are carbohydrates and a little bit of fat, but you're still completely eating predominantly carbohydrates that cause your blood sugar to rise and insulin to spike. Are you getting the picture? You're creating your own fatigue and you're creating it because you're eating way too many carbohydrates. The cycle can repeat itself over and over and over. It can go on all day long. **Download the Free companion PDF to this book at NoMoreFatigueextras.com.**

My Tamale Story

When I was new in practice, I had a very sweet patient who was always concerned about the fact that I didn't eat enough food. So one day when she came in for her treatment, she brought me a couple of tamales. That was very kind of her. I thought, "wow this is great." It was right before lunchtime, so I ate the tamales for lunch. Then I went back to work. I had a new patient. When I have new patients in my office, I do a consultation with them to find out what's wrong with them and ask all sorts of questions so that I am fully informed with what is going on with them and to build rapport. It's my time to shine, and first impressions are everything. Well, I'm in the middle of a consultation with this patient. While sitting across from her at my very wide antique desk, all of a sudden my eyelids, started to feel like a ton of bricks. I started to feel very uncomfortable, as I couldn't keep my eyelids open. This was not good because I'm in the middle of consulting with a brand-new patient. At this point, I am struggling and I'm thinking to myself that this can't be happening to me right now. I'm trying my best to continue the consultation, but my eyes are closing, and then my head dropped down and I kind of woke up as I was nodding off. This was horrible and absolutely unacceptable as you can imagine. I felt so embarrassed, and I couldn't believe it because this never happens. Suffice it to say the prospective new patient I had sitting in front of me never returned. I couldn't blame her. I'm sure she thought that I was rude and uncaring.

Proper Proportions

You need to eat your proteins, carbohydrates, and fats in the proper proportions to maximize energy and not spike your blood sugar and insulin levels. You need to have a 1 to 1 ratio of carbohydrates and protein and then have a 1/8 of the amount in good clean fats. The proper proportion is equivalent to one-part protein, one-part carbohydrate and one 1/8-part fat. So you look at the plate in front of you and half of the food should be protein and half should be a healthy, natural carbohydrate and about an 1/8 of good, clean fats. A healthy, natural carbohydrate is unprocessed or unrefined and what I'm recommending for you is a carbohydrate in the form of primarily vegetables and maybe a small potato, yam or a small portion of brown rice for that matter (although the portion sizes still work). For instance, if you're not going to eat vegetables, then I would not recommend half your plate with protein and half your plate with bread or pasta. For someone to make that piece of bread you want to eat or the pasta you're craving, they have to take a huge amount of grain and process it by blending it down to give you that bite sized roll. It's packed with calories and a super dense amount of carbohydrates, so the ration doesn't count as described above. If you're going to be eating a processed carb (bread, pasta) instead of whole unprocessed vegetables, potatoes, brown rice, then I would say eat 1-part protein and ½ a part bread or pasta (unless you're eating quinoa pasta which is high in protein) in order to keep the formula for increased energy from your meal.

My husband and I were invited to our friend's restaurant which was a panini shop. They're Italian and were having a special barbeque dinner after hours for a select few. I was worried that I was going to be fed lots of pasta, but they assured me that wouldn't be the case. I decided to go with my husband because he was super excited to go, and we also had some of our friends meeting us there. This place was an hour away from our home, and I made sure to pack my Tempurpedic transit pillow in the car, as I knew I would be sleeping on the way home. We arrived, and they were cooking the meat outside on a large square barbeque, and the meat had been cooking for many hours, I was told. We sat down to eat, and they had many courses that they brought out. We ate plate after plate after plate of delicious cuts of meat and sides of pasta, had wine, and even had homemade limoncello and a delicious cannoli for dessert, which we split (the best I've ever had). It was a fun evening, and I was so glad I went, and then we got into the car. I positioned the seat down so I could sleep and had my pillow under my neck so that my head wouldn't flail around while my husband drove us home. The funny thing that happened was that as we drove home, my husband and I carried on a conversation. I was wide awake. I couldn't believe it because I'm notorious for sleeping on the way home from dinner, even if it was only a mile or so away. It was so bizarre, I made a comment to my husband that the food must have been prepared with natural healthy ingredients and in the proper proportions because it was late and I wasn't tired at all despite the quantities I consumed that were well above my normal amount. This proves that when eaten in the right proportions, food can be nourishing and energizing for you without the fear of the dreaded food coma that happens when the blood sugar levels rise and insulin is spiked. When you're able to pair the protein with the carb and there is fiber present, your body will be able to gain sustained energy from the meal without the crash that normally occurs with simple refined sugars and empty calories that are consumed with junk food.

***

In my many years of reading countless books and trying all sorts new eating programs, I learned how to combine foods for maximum energy and metabolic burn. One of my favorite programs I purchased many years ago that stuck with me was called the *6 Week Body Makeover* or something like that. It was put out by Michael Thurmond, who was a personal trainer and appeared on the show *Extreme Makeover*, where they would take people who were unhappy with their appearance and transform them through plastic surgery and diet and exercise into "beautiful versions of themselves." They underwent drastic cosmetic surgery, diet and exercise programs, dental restorations, and even emotional therapy so that they would be happy with themselves. I purchased the program and went on to lose many pounds, getting to my high school weight at the end of the program. What I liked the most about the program was the fact that all the foods he recommended were natural and there were no processed foods. He recommended eating real food and not adding any sugar, salt, oils, or alcohol to meals. It fit well with my philosophy on which foods should be combined together and how much of each type should be consumed. It was scientifically based, and incorporated things I remember learning while in chiropractic school about metabolism and increasing your energy with food. Since then, I have moved on to different programs that work better for me, given my schedule, and for my husband, who did not like the foods that were recommended in that particular program. But I must say that when I eat, I always try to remember the way I learned to increase metabolic fire and boost my energy and metabolism as much as possible. The best thing is eating real foods that are not processed, eliminating bread, sugar, and added salt.

Cleansing Increases Energy

I have also done many different types of cleanses that I have enjoyed and have caused me to lose a few unwanted pounds, but most of all have doubled and tripled my energy levels. Sometimes my patients have asked me what the heck I was on because they saw me running around in my busy practice treating patients from room to room, not getting tired and being able to feel just as much energy at the end of the day as when I started. Some of the cleanses I recommended and coached my patients through were amazing for their health, but a bit difficult for many of them because it required they not eat any of the foods they wanted, only shakes and a few foods for twenty-one days of purification. Those that participated were very happy and did well, but I felt many were not able to follow the strict program.

Some people had sensitivities and food allergies, but craved the very foods that should have been eliminated. So at least with the twenty-one days of purification program, all food was eliminated and then reintroduced slowly so that they could see exactly which foods gave them the most difficulties. If you want to try an experiment on what foods are the most common in causing major fatigue and issues with health, you can eliminate the following: gluten, dairy, peanuts, corn, eggs, soy, and of course sugar (that includes artificial sweeteners). You can eliminate those for twenty-one days, and I can tell you that you will feel amazing. After the twenty-one days, you can reintroduce one food for one week and see how you feel. If all goes well and you feel great, then obviously that is not a problem food for you. You would repeat that again for another week and reintroduce a different food and see how it goes. You will know exactly which foods make you feel great, and which foods make you feel like crap. If the foods do not agree with you, then they become those you should avoid. Most of the foods you will not want to give up are the foods you shouldn't be eating, and you will see your energy and productivity go through the roof once they are eliminated from your diet.

You may think there is no way you can do this, but I promise you that you absolutely can. In the meantime, you can substitute coconut milk for milk, eat quinoa pasta for regular pasta, and coconut aminos for those of you that need to eat soy. Many years ago, I substituted almonds for peanuts, and I've never gone back. I used to be one of those people that ate peanut butter out of the jar, but I have been buying almond butter for at least twenty years, if not longer, and yes, I eat it out of the jar. In the case of sugar, you may say it would be horrible to go through your life without it, but I'm here to tell you that if it harms you and zaps your energy, then you should remove it from the foods you eat. Remember, if it's your birthday and you want to eat cake, then do it and have a great time, but don't make the mistake of living your life without energy and vitality over sugar because you're stubborn and want to eat it every day. Do yourself a favor and treat your body like a temple and be good to it, and it will be good to you! Listen to your body and try out different ways of eating. I promise you that you will find a way that works for you if it is your true desire to be healthy and to have energy in your life. Remember if you eat good, clean, and healthy foods, you're going to have better sleep and when you sleep well you have more energy!

My Favorite Cleanse

My favorite cleanse is the Isagenix system. I absolutely love it and have been on it for over 10 years. It is basically combining protein shakes with a sensible meal along with intermittent fasting for 10-48 hours depending on my mood and willpower. The protein shakes help to nourish me quickly when I don't have time to eat. With the sensible meals, I try to always make it a Michael Thurmond type of meal in the proper proportion. I like the system and have tweaked it a bit over the years to my liking so that I get the best results in energy.

In the toxic world we live in, it is important to perpetually do nutritional cleanses so that we detoxify our cells and tissues so that we can be healthy and feel great! It's like taking a shower or brushing your teeth. You wouldn't go two weeks without either one of those, I hope.

***

The new craze that I've been hearing all about recently is intermittent fasting, which requires you to fast for extended periods of time each and every day, such as waiting to eat your first meal (or only meal) at noon and eating higher fat and protein type meals for about a six to eight-hour feeding window (sometimes longer). I see some value in that, but I like to combine the different methods in my own customized way of eating for health, energy, and productivity. I will say that when my husband went to visit his family back in Denmark, and I was left home alone to fend for myself, I tried to eat a modified intermittent fasting type of way and I liked it. I had my shake for breakfast around 11 or 12 noon, and then I would have a salad (I purchased those premade salads from Trader Joes) with chicken around 4 or 5pm, then I would fast the rest of the day. I felt good and I was able to eat like that for the two weeks he was gone without any issues. I haven't stuck with that, per se, but I have tried to eat my breakfast shake as late in the morning as possible, and then I always like to not eat within three to four hours of sleep.

Another thing that has worked for me which I also recommend is keeping a food journal so you are mindfully aware of what you put in your mouth every second of every day. It's amazing how you don't remember everything that you're consuming on a daily basis unless you're writing it down. As an added bonus, it helps you not only remember, it sometimes helps you put off those snacks and eat better because you don't want to write it down. It also makes it super easy to portion your meals better, too, because you're writing down your portions.

One last thing I highly recommend is for you to stop snacking all day long, as that will zap your energy (your body will constantly be having to use energy to digest food instead of doing all the projects or exercise you want to be doing), and you don't really need the food. That's what is called emotional eating or boredom. You should eat when you're hungry, not when you're bored or emotional or any other time. You may need to ask yourself when you walk into the pantry and you're looking for food, "Am I really hungry?", "When was the last time I ate?", "Can I wait until my next meal?" If it's late at night, ask yourself, "when do I plan to go to bed," and "am I leaving at least three to four hours of fasting before bedtime?" These are some of the action steps you can take to help you stay on track, and if you absolutely, positively have to eat something at night after dinner and you know you can't help it, then have a ½-1 cup of berries (I love raspberries or blueberries) as an evening snack, as it won't spike your blood sugar too badly, and the antioxidants are good for you.

I hope you have a better understanding of how eating the right foods in the right proportions at the right times is critical to feeling great and being super productive. It is really easy to do (and easy not to do). The choice is yours. I have coached thousands of patients with this, and it's not that hard to implement. The changes in energy are staggering when you follow the recommendations and combine your foods properly (protein and carbs in a 1:1 ratio, and add clean healthy fats - 1/8 part). Remember, this is a great way to easily boost your energy. Be mindful of what you're eating, and don't forget the blood sugar/insulin spikes and how detrimental that can be for your overall energy. Talk to your doctor before making any changes to your health and eating routine.

Chapter 5

What's so Important About Water?

Drinking the right amount and type of water, and knowing when to drink water is critical to feeling great and being super productive in everything you do. You should pour yourself a glass of water as you read this chapter. It's very important for you to understand. Most people don't drink enough water, and you absolutely need water for health and wellbeing because we are made of about 60% water, and we need to replenish the water we lose every day in order to perform our bodily functions. Our muscles are about 80% water, and our blood is about 90% water.

I met a woman that never drank water, and I didn't understand how she could survive without it. She looked fairly healthy from the outside and even worked out, but she did not drink water. What I found out later was that she had a lot of health issues and suffered from severe fatigue and various other health problems. I'm not sure if this is because of her lack of water consumption, but she was never able to have kids and what looked like a beautiful woman on the outside did not equate to a healthy person on the inside. Water is essential if you're going to be truly healthy. Drinking plenty of water increases your energy levels, helps you look younger and better, drastically improves your mental clarity, and helps detoxify your body.

Water helps to deliver oxygen all over the body through the blood. It helps get rid of the sludge in your body by improving your lymphatic drainage and keeps you hydrated as you expel toxins through your skin and bowel and bladder. Besides feeling great, you can look great and have beautiful skin because staying hydrated plumps your skin and gives you a younger look. Have you ever seen anyone that looks much younger than they were because they had beautiful skin? It goes the other way, too. Dehydration ages your skin, and you look much older.

Consumption of Water

In order to feel great and function well, you need to drink half your body weight in ounces. If you weigh 140 pounds, then that means you need to drink 70 ounces of water every day to function at optimum levels and to feel energized. If you put water in a coffee maker and drink the coffee that comes out, then that does not count for the amount of water for your day. Coffee is very dehydrating to the body and if you need 70 ounces of water per day and you drink 12 ounces of coffee the same day then you would have to replenish for the extra 12 ounces of coffee. Therefore, if you weigh 140 pounds then you would have to consume 70 + 12 ounces of water total, making it a total of 82 ounces per day. There are a couple of times where this formula can change and you may need a bit more water, and that is when it is extremely hot out and you're exercising a lot. Don't wait until you feel thirsty, because if you do, then that means you are already dehydrated and chronic dehydration compromises your overall health, wellness, and wellbeing because our cells cannot function well if they are dried up.

When to Drink Water

Now that you know you need to drink water to improve your energy and vitality, it is best to drink it away from meals. I recommend you consume 16 ounces of water upon awakening and then another 16 ounces thirty to sixty minutes before eating your meals, and you should also have a glass of water (8 ounces) right before bedtime. This will keep your body functioning optimally and help with detoxification and also helps build your energy levels. This is one of the easiest steps because it is something you can start doing right now.

I had a friend that was an avid cyclist and she did not like to drink much water. She said she didn't think it was that important. She was out on a long ride with some friends, and she just keeled over completely dehydrated and felt dizzy and weak, then her legs started cramping. Not getting enough water and fluids leads to dehydration and that will detrimentally affect your quality of life. You will feel fatigued all the time. When you're drinking plenty of water, your blood stays thin, but if you are not, that leads to dehydration and you get thicker blood, and it causes your heart to have to work harder, and that causes you to feel fatigue and brain fog and even causes headaches.

Water is important for proper elimination of toxins through the kidneys and colon. When you don't drink enough water, you will get constipated. That lack of proper elimination can cause you to retain and reabsorb the toxins you should be eliminating, zapping your energy and making you feel sick. Drink that water and get that poop out of there so you can feel energized again. And if we're talking about elimination, let me tell you that the less water you drink, the less you pee and the less you pee causes you to be predisposed to kidney stones as the minerals build up in your urine, and this of course is worsened by drinking too much coffee and consuming too much salt. Save yourself a lot of grief and drink more water! In fact, not drinking enough water can stress your liver. The liver's job is to filter out your toxins. Again, it's easier for it to work when your blood is thin, and that happens when you're getting adequate water.

Now that you know the formula, you should really know whether you're drinking enough water or not. But if that doesn't convince you, then be aware that signs of dehydration include thirst (once you get thirsty, you're already dehydrated, so don't wait to be thirsty) and dry mouth (this happens when you've been drinking). Alcohol is a diuretic, so drink a glass of water between drinks and before going to bed. If you haven't been drinking water and have headaches and dry skin and feel dizzy or light-headed and cannot pee, that should give you a clue as well, so grab a bottle of water and drink up.

Alkaline Water

There's a difference between regular water and alkaline water. Normal drinking water has a neutral PH of 7. Alkaline water has higher PH levels. I personally drink Kangen water 9.5 PH level. I drink alkaline water as much as possible because I want to neutralize the acid in my body. Diseases from an acidic environment can arise, so you might want to become more alkaline and that can be accomplished by eating lots of alkaline foods, like deep, green, leafy vegetables instead of meat, fish, and eggs. Alkaline foods help you to treat and prevent various medical conditions like heart disease, diabetes, osteoarthritis, and cancer.

Many people don't want to eat foods that are classified as alkaline because they don't like vegetables, so they opt in to drink the water which is easy and tasty. Kangen water goes through an electrolysis process and makes the water molecules smaller (microclusters) because the process splits the water molecule, making it very easy to swallow and be absorbed inside your cells, improving your hydration. When you drink regular water, it can sometimes sit inside your stomach and make you feel bloated, but with these microclusters, they easily enter the cells because they are so small. I can personally drink a lot more Kangen water than regular water because it doesn't sit in my stomach. It is easily absorbed in my body.

The bottom line is you need to drink the correct amount of water in order to have the vitality and energy to help you to feel great and be super productive in everything you do.

Chapter 6

Nutritional Supplements That Matter

I have been asked many times whether it's really that important to take vitamins and minerals or if it's okay to just eat healthy, balanced meals. I have studied this quite a bit, and I must note the difference in our food's nutritional values today as compared to when my dad was a kid in the mid-1940s. If you were to eat a bowl of salad back then and compare it to a bowl of salad now, there is a stark difference in the nutritional value of that bowl of salad. You might ask how many bowls of salad would you have to eat today in order to have the same nutritional value of a bowl of salad back then. The answer might shock you. You would have to eat around 20 bowls of salad. The reason why is that our soils are depleted of their nutritional value due to over farming and lack of minerals. The foods we eat do not have the same nutritional value they once had. Then on top of that, we cook our foods and over process them, depleting the nutritional value again. It is too hard to get all the nutrition we need if we depend on getting all the nutrients our bodies need through our foods alone. I can tell you that the body is miraculous and it can keep on going despite poor nutrition, but to really thrive and consume all the nutrients we need for great health and lots of energy, we do need to supplement. We would need to eat truckloads of food, and there is no way we are going to eat truckloads of food in order to get all the nutrients we need to carry out all the important processes our bodies are involved in every minute of every day.

Basic Nutritional Supplements

There are many different types of supplements and it is super hard to figure out exactly what we need when the choices are vast, and the different brands are numerous. You get what you pay for, so a good quality multivitamin and multimineral is essential as a start. Make sure you are taking vitamin D. Even though you can get vitamin D from the sun, in order to get it from the sun we need 20 minutes of full body exposure every single day. That does not happen especially in the winter or if you're indoors a lot or use sunscreen. Vitamin D will be in a multivitamin, but maybe not at the right amount. I recommend you take at least 4000-8000 IU per day. However, it is a good idea to get your levels checked because not everyone absorbs it well. The optimum functional levels should be 50-80. If your levels are between 20-50 then you are considered somewhat deficient and should take even more in order to get those levels to the optimum as mentioned above.

Vitamin K2 is essential for the proper utilization of vitamin D. Vitamin K2 sources come from eggs, butter, and dairy that come from happy, grass-fed cows, fermented foods, and certain cheeses like brie and gouda. In order to increase brain function vitamin D, tryptophan, and omega 3 are needed together to increase concentration of brain serotonin without any side effects. Omega 3s come from salmon, sardines, mackerel, and anchovies. Omega 3s are critical for increased brain function, while low levels of DHA is linked to many brain degenerative conditions like depression, memory loss, and Alzheimer's dementia.

You should also make sure you are not deficient in magnesium, as it helps with chronic fatigue as well as viral infections and many other illnesses. Unfortunately, most of us are deficient in magnesium. Many of the vitamins we take such as calcium, vitamin K2, and vitamin D must be balanced with magnesium in order for them to work properly. Magnesium is necessary to activate muscles and nerves, create energy in the body by activating ATP, help us digest macronutrients, and it's as a precursor for neurotransmitters like serotonin, the feel-good hormone. Magnesium is found in bananas, avocados, nuts, spinach. A magnesium deficiency leads to unexplained fatigue and chronic fatigue, weakness in the body, hormone imbalances, depression, anxiety, fibromyalgia, musculoskeletal conditions, headaches and much, much more. You can always supplement multivitamin/multiminerals with specific vitamins to help with challenges in life like trouble sleeping, and health challenges from your heart, stomach, or bones.

Materials vs. Labor

Vitamins and minerals give our bodies the basic building blocks or materials to make our structure. If you think of our body like a house, then we need these building blocks like a home needs wood for the frame and cement and drywall and stone for the floor or countertops, nails, glue, etc. We need the basic materials for our house. You don't want to build your body with paper towels instead of bricks or trash instead of cement do you? We need to eat well and take high quality vitamins and minerals so that we can build a strong and healthy energetic body. It is important to supplement with vitamins and minerals.

Plant antioxidants help us with the effects of oxidative stress on our bodies. While I have always been a proponent of taking plant antioxidants, recently I discovered that, with the right building blocks in our body and the right cellular function, we can make our own natural antioxidants that, in most cases, are overwhelmingly stronger than plant antioxidants.

Remember the show that was on television called *Extreme Makeover: Home Edition*? It was about helping families with their home needs due to the horrible living conditions they had. For the homeowner, maybe they had mold growing in some places and a family member was sick, or maybe it was a veteran that needed help, or maybe it was a family that was living in unsafe conditions, or the house was too small, etc. Either way, they found a small dilapidated home and rebuilt it in one week while the family went on vacation. These homes went from a tiny, nonfunctional home to a beautiful and functional home in just one week. The way they were able to transform these homes was to have a crew of thousands of workers and then have all the materials they needed at the job site and have thousands of people around the clock ready, willing, and able to do the job. They had inspectors and foremen all working together to build the beautiful home.

There is something similar happening with regard to your body being tired and fatigued. We all need the right materials for our body, and we also need the labor, too. What would happen if, on the home makeover show, they had all the right materials that were needed for the build but only five people showed up to work? It's not going to get done in a week. What would happen if they did not have the blueprints available? Or maybe they did not have the general contractor or foreman telling the workers what to do? The work would not get done properly. What if a thousand people showed up on the job site, but no materials or the wrong materials were available for the job? It's not going to go well. How does this compare to our bodies?

We need all the building blocks, macros and micros, in order to build a beautiful, healthy, and energized body, then we need the blueprints and labor to get the job done. We need workers, plumbers, electricians, framers, tile layers, floor installers, inspectors, project managers, designers etc. in our body also along with the blueprints that tell these laborers how to put all the materials into our bodies (our house) properly and to the right code.

Redox Signaling Molecules

The labor that is used by the body are directed by these little molecules called redox signaling molecules. These little molecules are the labor, and they are signaling molecules that can message the rest of the body like an inspector telling an electrician that they need to move the outlet to a different wall, or what to do to make sure the house is being built properly and safely so that there won't be any issues later. These molecules are made by the mitochondria, the cellular engines in each of our cells. Without these little molecules, we would die. When we are young, our bodies make these molecules in abundant numbers, but as we age, the numbers fall greatly, and that is what determines how we function and if we age gracefully or not.

Remember when we were kids? We could play all day long and run around and never get tired, and we would have boundless energy that never seems to end. We would wake up the next day ready to do it again and again and again. We never complained that we had back pain or our bodies hurt. We were kids. Kids burn free fatty acids instead of muscle glycogen like adults, so they have more energy and don't get sore in the process. Adults primarily burn muscle glycogen, so when we do things and exert our bodies we get sore and ache all over and get super tired too. When we have damage to our cells, the body is supposed to detect that damage quickly and take care of it by either signaling to our body that the cell needs to be repaired, if that's possible, or if it's too damaged, then the cell needs to be replaced. That is exactly what happens when our bodies function well and we have all the building blocks and labor to get it done. When we don't have the necessary building blocks or the workers that do the labor don't show up for work or don't understand what to do because of a weak cell signal, then we have problems.

How We Make Energy

We have about 75 trillion cells in our body and they all have a nucleus and lots of mitochondria (100-2000 depending on the type of cell) and other organelles. The cell membrane has gaps in it and allows some things to enter and keeps other things out. The mitochondria represent the cellular engines, power houses, or battery packs of each cell. Most of our energy comes from the ATP produced by the mitochondria. The nucleus contains DNA and sends signals into the cell to assure the cell performs the required functions as well as any maintenance and detoxification necessary for longevity. For instance, when we eat carbs, it is broken down into simple sugars like glucose, and this enters the cell through the cell membrane, and it enters into the mitochondria, and this then becomes part of the energy cycle. As this occurs in the mitochondria, energy is produced and redox signaling molecules are also produced in equal parts as a byproduct. We have reductants and oxidants in equal parts, hence the name redox. These molecules are responsible for regulating all the chemical reactions that occur in our bodies. It was not until recently that the importance of these redox signaling molecules was discovered. **Download the Free companion PDF to this book at NoMoreFatigueextras.com.**

Army (Oxidants) and the Shield (Reductants)

Oxidants represents the army which help the immune system, and it basically targets external threats like viruses, or bacteria to the cells. The reductants represent the shield, and they activate antioxidant production due to internal threats. The main thing you have to know is that if the army and shield are in perfect balance, then the cell is healthy. A healthy cell not only functions properly, but can eliminate the things that shouldn't be in the cell. The shield creates protective enzymes and helps the cell so that the army doesn't destroy the good things. When our cells get damaged, they show too much of the army, and there is not enough shield to protect the organelles, so this can create damage on the mitochondria and on the DNA. All health problems can be linked to damaged cells. If we can repair or replace damaged cells more effectively we can minimize the effects of aging, injury or disease.

Oxidative Stress and Antioxidants

Oxidative stress is a primary contributor to hundreds of health challenges. There are many things that cause oxidative stress like mental stress, excessive or no exercise, inadequate hydration, cigarette smoke, lack of proper nutrition, prescription medications, negative mental attitude, electromagnetic radiation, ultraviolet radiation, pollution, food additives and preservatives, insecticides, pesticides, herbicides, toxic chemicals, and the list goes on and on. There have been thousands of toxic chemicals dumped into our environment over the years, and this is causing us to struggle with our health and make it impossible to have the energy we need to get through the day. We are exposed to more chemical pollutants in 15 minutes today than our great-great-grandparents were exposed in their entire lives. Many of the chemicals were synthesized by mankind and our ancestors were never before exposed to them. This causes huge challenges to our immune system in determining how to react to these new exposures found in the air we breathe, the food we eat, and the water we drink. These chemicals are free radicals and they are harming us.

How do we eliminate free radical damage? With natural antioxidants made inside our cells! I have been taking plant antioxidants for years in order to eliminate the free radicals that I have in my body, but recently learned that it is impossible to eliminate these free radicals with plant antioxidants alone because there are 100 sextillion free radicals created in our body every single day. We would have to eat truckloads of plant antioxidants in order to keep up, and that's just not going to happen. Unfortunately, these antioxidants are too large to pass through the cell membrane. It's like trying to throw a basketball at a chain link fence and expecting it to pass through. It can't pass through, and these large antioxidants cannot pass through our cell membrane either. If all health challenges are linked to damaged cells, then how are we going to be able increase our antioxidant defenses to fix these damaged cells if the plant antioxidants can't pass through the cell membrane? We are not going to be able to with plant antioxidants! That's the problem here, and that's one of the reasons we are not able to help our body become healthy and vibrant like we want it to be purely with plant antioxidants. Plant antioxidants can clean up the free radicals at about a ratio of 1:1 which means for every plant antioxidant we would be able to eliminate 1 free radical. The problem is that we have way too many free radicals as mentioned above…100 sextillion! When I first learned this, I was disappointed with the fact that I had thought I was doing such a great job consuming these plant antioxidants that were not making a dent in combating all the free radicals I was being exposed to. It was quite depressing.

However, there is some good news, these redox signaling molecules that are produced in our body by our mitochondria are available as a supplement that can and will increase the production of intracellular antioxidants and they are far more effective as you will see below.

My Accident Nightmare

I found this out after having a bad auto accident where a big Yukon XL plowed into the back of my car. It felt like I got hit with a baseball bat in the back of my head, and then the seatbelt retracted, pinning me to the seat while I felt like the wind got knocked out of me. I had a burn across my chest from the seatbelt, and I was clearly shaken by the crash. Instantly, I felt a brain fog come over me and I felt confused. I was lucky to be alive, but my body was in bad shape. My brain was having problems thinking. I instantly felt depressed about it and my energy levels that were normally quite high had plummeted. The pain in my neck and back was pretty bad, and I couldn't sit at my computer to do any paperwork for any length of time without having to stop. I was struggling just to get through my day and had no energy for anything. My pain persisted and was worse with any movement and, of course, sitting in front of the computer, which luckily, I did not do much of. My paperwork piled up as I could not do much, and the situation got really bad.

My chiropractor and I decided I should have an MRI to see what else was going on because I wasn't getting any better. I got the results of the MRIs and found out why I was in so much pain and why it wasn't going away. What left me scared to death, however, was that the MRI also showed lesions in my liver and right kidney. Hearing that news, my heart sank. I was already feeling horrible from the injuries I incurred from the accident, and now this news freaked me out. Immediately I thought to myself, do I have cancer? Why would I have lesions in my liver and kidney? It was a scary time. The radiologist recommended I have another MRI. This time, it would scan my abdomen with contrast dye to evaluate it further. It seems like I instantly went into a deep depression and felt exhausted and terrified about what they might find. The day after my MRI, I was supposed to get together with a dear friend, a holistic health practitioner that was in town for her son's wedding, and I didn't want to tell anyone about what I was going through. Quite frankly, I just couldn't even talk about it without breaking down emotionally. She knew I had had an accident, and I told her that I was in pain. I told my husband we would go to dinner, but not to mention anything about the other findings because I wasn't ready to talk about it. I was too emotional and I didn't want to break down in a restaurant. We had a nice dinner, and while we were eating, she shared with me that she and her husband were working with several doctors across the country using redox signaling molecules.

Redox Signaling Molecules

I frankly had never heard of these redox signaling molecules and had a hard time understanding them, but learned they help the body work better and help with the healing process by turning on the genes, and I should try them in addition to everything else I was doing. I agreed because I thought, "Well, what do I have to lose? It would be great if it could help me with my pain, and it could not hurt." She gave me a topical gel containing these redox signaling molecules, which I applied to my neck and upper back. That seemed to help. It actually decreased some of the spasm and pain in my neck as I sat in the booth. The following day, I learned that there was a drink that contained the molecules as well as the topical gel. I decided to drink the liquid and apply the gel topically. It helped. I started researching these little molecules because, as a doctor, I wanted to learn the mechanism of action, and I learned a lot. I learned that the more redox signaling molecules you have in your body, the better it functions. We have large numbers of these molecules as kids, but then the numbers rapidly decrease over time.

The good news is that even if I didn't have a large quantity of these molecules any more due to my age, I could supplement to bring those levels up. Luckily the molecules are tiny in size, about three to four atoms, which allows them to get absorbed into our cells unlike the plant antioxidants that are about 200 molecules in size. It's like if we were throwing marbles at the chain link fence. They will be able to get through. These little redox molecules can also cross the blood brain barrier and enter inside our brain cells, and enter inside the mitochondria and even into the nucleus. Redox signaling molecules trigger the production of natural antioxidants inside our cells. These signaling molecules quickly disperse throughout the body and immediately go to work in our body where ever they're needed. They communicate within and between our cells in order to restore function and facilitate cellular repair. I can tell you that my thinking got better and my energy went up, but most of all, I had hope after learning all about it that this could help me no matter what my body was battling.

Glutathione, the Mother of All Antioxidants

As a chiropractor, I have been teaching my patients for over 30 years that the body heals itself. Learning more about the effects of these little molecules was in total alignment with everything I believed in, and I wasn't scared any more. I just wanted to give my body a boost to allow it to heal as quickly and completely as possible, and I wanted to keep learning more and more about how this could help me to heal. A natural antioxidant is made inside our own cells instead of a plant derived one that we consume. The effectiveness of natural Glutathione to clean up our cells from free radicals is about 70 million free radicals cleaned up and neutralized per every one natural antioxidant every second of every day. The more I learned about this, the more excited I got! It's amazing that we can supplement these redox signaling molecules and that they can get inside our cells and go to the right cells that are damaged to clean and detoxify them quickly and effectively. Glutathione is considered the most important antioxidant you need to stay healthy. It's considered the mother of all antioxidants. We lose around 15% of it for every decade we're alive, starting at about age twenty. Therefore, as we age, we have lower and lower levels of glutathione. Studies show that 80 percent of people hospitalized with chronic illnesses have a glutathione deficiency. I had heard of a few friends trying to increase their levels of glutathione by taking it orally or injecting it. But I learned when researching it that if it is taken orally it gets destroyed in the digestive tract and can't be absorbed by the body readily due to its size, and if given intravenously, the molecules are so large they cannot get inside the cells.

Jean Carper, who is a leading authority on health and nutrition and bestselling author of numerous books on health and aging, stated that "you must get your levels of glutathione up if you want to keep your youth and live longer. High levels of glutathione predict good health as you age and a long life. Low levels predict early disease and death."

Proper Dosing of Redox Signaling Molecules

You can supplement your own production of natural intracellular glutathione with redox cell signaling molecules. These molecules will increase the glutathione production and activity within our cells by 500-800%. As we supplement with these tiny molecules, they help our cells perform the required functions as well as any maintenance and detoxification necessary for longevity. If you're under forty years old, I recommend 2 ounces twice per day and if you're over fifty, I recommend 4 ounces twice a day. These doses are a good rule for a maintenance dose when all is well and you want it to stay that way, but if, at any time, you have health challenges and want to supplement with this so that the body has an added boost to allow it to heal up faster, I recommend you double or triple the dose depending on the severity of the situation. Once I started taking this for my accident, I took 2 ounces twice a day for about three days, then I doubled it to 4 ounces twice a day, and then I tripled it until I was able to get my pain under control. I also wanted to take a bit extra due to my liver and kidney issues. I can say that it did make me feel better and helped me think better and gave me the energy I needed to get through my day. Luckily for me, the further testing and visit to a GI specialist confirmed the lesions they found in my kidney and liver were simple cysts. I am very relieved it was not something more serious, but still don't understand why I had that in the first place. I continue to take my redox signaling molecules as well as my vitamins, minerals, herbal extracts, 16 probiotic strains, and three kinds of prebiotic fiber that feeds the friendly bacteria and antioxidants. My energy level has gone up and stayed consistently high since. So now you know that you have to supplement with vitamins and minerals and I'm happy to have introduced some of you to redox signaling molecules that have been working in your own body to help you function and heal on a cellular level. You know that they are produced by the mitochondria inside each of your cells, and you can supplement to increase the level to what you once had when you were a kid.

What Doesn't Kill Us Makes Us Stronger

As we age, the numbers of mitochondria are reduced in our body. We can naturally increase the number and size of mitochondria and indirectly increase the production of energy in our body by a process called hormesis. This process puts a mild acute stress on our body, causing it to adapt and get stronger and healthier in more ways than one. This, in turn, increases the size and number of our cells' power houses, the mitochondria discussed above. I am not talking about severe stress nor chronic exposure here. A healthy person can expose their body to mild acute stress levels in the following ways: increased exercise, intermittent fasting, cold exposure, heat exposure, hypoxia from being at altitudes, oxygen deprivation as in holding our breath under water (don't try to win the Guinness world record), prolonged sun exposure, dietary phytochemicals. The key is starting slowly. The increased energy can be double or triple what you have now because of the increased number and size of the mitochondria in your cells. It occurs by introducing a stressor as mentioned above and as a result the body increases its resistance to other stressors, making it healthier and more resilient.

Use It or Lose It

Mitochondria are like muscles, they shrink when they are not used and grow when they are used. You can exercise more and as you get fitter and stronger naturally, those little power houses in your muscle cells will increase in number and size, and as that happens, you will naturally have a greater production in your body. Remember the mitochondria are the power houses in your cells, and you are made up of cells, so you will have more energy. We'll talk about exercise below, but in the context of increasing your mitochondrial size and number, you will have to do exercises that stretch you and create more strength and stamina, which would be cardiovascular exercise that gets longer and harder over time mixed with weight resistance exercise to pump up the volume in your muscles. You get the picture! Work out harder and longer to challenge your body to keep growing and improving. Don't want to keep doing the same things that don't keep pushing you.

Cold Exposure

Another way of increasing your mitochondrial size and number is to shock your body a bit and put stress on it like cold showers or cold baths or swimming in the cold. This will build your mitochondrial size and numbers. If you're going to try this method, I suggest you start with the warm shower first and end with the cold. This is easier. Believe me, I tried it, and it is tough going into a cold shower first thing in the morning, but do it, if possible. When I first learned this method, I thought of jumping into my cold pool in the deep end and having to swim to the shallow end to get out. I was all gung-ho about it and thought I definitely wanted to increase my mitochondrial size and numbers. How many times did I do this? Well, let me tell you that I couldn't bring myself to doing it even once. Maybe in the summer time but not in winter. I still have the intention, but I haven't brought myself to do it because there is a better way. Drinking the molecules sounds better to me, but if you want an invigorating experience that will wake you up and energize you and build your cellular engine, then by all means, cold water exposure is a good way.

We talked about water in the last chapter, and actually drinking water first thing in the morning and before bed time allows you to naturally build these little power houses, too. They naturally build at night when you're sleeping and away from your eating window. There is always a reason for my recommendations.

To the question of "do you need to supplement?" The answer is *yes*! You need to take a high-quality multivitamin and multimineral at the very least.

Gut Health

You need to feed your gut too. You feed your gut with probiotics (try to consume as many different strains as possible), which increase the numbers of the good and healthy bacteria that help you with digestion because they optimize the repopulation of beneficial bacteria in the intestinal tract. And I believe you need to feed those little guys with prebiotics also so they can be healthy and keep you healthy and energized as well. The enteric nervous system is known as your second brain because it can operate independently of the central nervous system, and it's true when you think that our amazing body lives off what we feed it. Be good to your body and it will be good to you.

***

To recap, eat a healthy diet and take a multivitamin and multimineral so that your body has all the building blocks ready to build or rebuild or repair your house, take a probiotic that includes a prebiotic so that all the food and supplements you take are bioavailable to you and aren't just passing through you. It's not going to help you if it's not assimilated into your body. Then you need the labor (redox signaling molecules) to help your cells read the blueprints and know where to repair or replace your tissues when they get damaged and to help keep you functioning like a machine on a cellular level. If your cells are healthy, then your tissues are healthy, and if your tissues are healthy, then your organs are healthy, and if your organs are healthy, you are healthy. A healthy body is an energized body.

You can increase your number and size of the mitochondria which is the production plants of these little molecules, or you can supplement. Personally, I try to do both because I know the numbers are diminishing with age and oxidative stress, and I want to keep the redox signaling molecules balanced and as high as possible so I can function like I did when I was a kid. At the very least, I supplement with these molecules. I have used these molecules for many patients in my office and the results have been staggering. I can tell you that I have had patients with lethargy and other issues that had disappeared, and the most incredible thing has been the speed at which that has happened.

When you have all the materials you need (vitamins and minerals), and you have all the labor you need (redox signaling molecules), and you can read the blueprints

(DNA), and can communicate clearly (did I mention redox signaling molecules are like actual cellphones that communicate, hence the name signaling) every step of the way on how to do it, then you have a wonderful finished product. This is how you can create that extreme makeover right inside your own body and why it happens so rapidly. You want lots of materials for your remodel with lots of laborers ready to work with good plans, with foremen and inspectors to make sure it's done right.

Do yourself a favor and make sure you give your body everything it needs so that you can stay healthy if you are well or get healthy if you have a health challenge. If you're not able to live your life to the fullest, everything suffers. I hope you now understand just how important it is to eat healthy and to supplement with vitamins, minerals, and redox signaling molecules in order to feel great and be super productive at work. These supplements are not intended to diagnose, treat, or cure any disease or health condition.

Chapter 7

Good Night and Sleep Tight

"Take rest; a field that has rested
gives a bountiful crop."
– Ovid

S leep is the number one longevity factor and is
very important with regards to energy levels.
Everyone knows that when you don't get a good
night's sleep, then you are tired and grumpy the next
day. There's a difference between rest and sleep, and
it should really matter to you. You need seven to eight
hours of uninterrupted sleep every single night. Uninterrupted because the most important kind of sleep is
restorative sleep, which is deep sleep or REM (rapid eye
movement) sleep when you're vividly dreaming. It takes

a while to cycle into that type of sleep. Even though you may be vividly dreaming, the body is relaxed almost like if it were paralyzed. Different levels of sleep rest the brain and rest the body. Sleeping 7-8 hours allows your body to go through all the different stages of sleep and allow for maximum rejuvenation and rest and healing. So if you go to sleep and sleep a couple hours and get up to go to the bathroom, then fall asleep again, and then your husband's snoring wakes you up a couple hours later, and then you fall asleep again and a neighbor's dog barks, and then you try to sleep but now you can't for a half hour or so, and then you hear the hustle and bustle of cars driving on their way to work, and then the alarm goes off and it's time to get up and start your day, then you did not get enough restorative sleep due to waking up every few hours.

Your body needs the rest, and light sleeping is not adequate for health reasons. Sleep is when your body and mind cease to function consciously or voluntarily. Rest is not sleep. It is just when you cease from effort or activity for a period of time. Short periods of rest throughout the day is beneficial, but at night you should be sleeping so that you can cycle through the sleep stages and truly benefit.

Rest

We all need to take short periods of rest throughout our day, and when you think about it, it can be just the break you need when the stress starts to build. Many of us are so busy that we don't have the time to take a break and don't want to stop what we're doing. I can say I have been guilty of that myself too many times. Deadlines aren't going to be accomplished while we are taking a break, and I want to tell you that I have found that, with myself and my patients, productivity goes way down as you keep going without a break, so think of it as rebooting your computer so that you can get more done and get it done quicker. I like to recommend that you take a few breaks throughout the day that last about 3-5 minutes at a time, just to rest your brain and reset your stress. I do deep breathing and like to induce a few yawns, as I heard that will lower any stress you are experiencing at the same time. I recommend that you take 3-5 breaks lasting 3-5 minutes. When you do that, you will feel better right away and your productivity will increase instantly.

A Variation of Rest

I have had several people that just refuse to take a break and rest because of time and deadlines. So I have modified it in two ways which I feel still make a huge impact on stress and productivity. Since most of my patients and clients are sitting at a computer, I have them do a stretch every 20 minutes or so that only lasts about 15-20 seconds. This resets their posture and mind at the same time. I have them look up as far as possible while they open the chest and squeeze their shoulder blades together gently. They do this for 15-20 seconds while they breathe in deeply 2-3 times or induce a yawn. This resets their posture and brain and alleviates some of the tension that develops in the neck and shoulders and upper back. This allows you to take a short break and rest your mind and body and reset your posture, which are necessary. Try this if you are too busy to take the longer rest periods where you close your eyes for 3-5 minutes while breathing deeply and feeling grateful for being alive. This has been so beneficial for so many people, and I believe it will be for you as well.

Last Variation

Many of my high-powered executive clients want to take a break but just get too involved with their work, so if they are unable to take the small breaks mentioned above, I give them this last variation. You can do this at the very least since you want to increase your energy and productivity. Set an alarm or mindfulness clock to chime in at the top of the hour, and when it does, open the chest by bringing your arms out at about a 45 degree to your sides palms forward and simultaneously taking your head backward like you are looking up at the ceiling, but as far back as possible behind you, and hold that and breathe deeply, slowly and focus your breath or yawn. Hold this position for 30 to 60 seconds.

Charge Up the Break with a Short Meditation or Affirmation

I like to add thoughts like, "thank you God for the many blessings in my life," or "I am so happy and grateful now that I have_____" (you fill in the blank), "every day in every way, I'm feeling better and better," "I am well and I am energized today and every day in order to do everything I need to do and more." You get the picture. Do this every hour at the top of the hour. You'd be surprised to know how much energy you will have to get the job done. And you will be doing it with gratitude, for your life is richer and more fulfilling than if you were concentrating on your work. You might say you don't have the time to do this, but I challenge you to do it anyway and see just how much more productive you are when you start practicing this. As a side benefit, the posture stretch will allow your body to reset itself so you don't end up looking like the hunchback from Notre Dame. We all have a minute at the top of the hour, and if you can make this a habit, you'll be glad you did as your work productivity, posture, and fulfilment in life will go up. So remember to take these short breaks like you're powering down your mind and body, and feel fresh and rejuvenated at work. If someone asks what you're doing, share this with them, too. I think too many of us forget to take a short break for mental and physical wellbeing so that we can be, do, and have more in our lives, and we can achieve more as well.

Your body and your mind will thank you for the care you give it. Remember, this is the body you get to live in for the rest of your life, and I recommend you treat it like it were your precious child, with love and self-care. If you do this daily while at work, I promise you will be more productive, more energized, and happier too.

Circadian Rhythm

When you get home and you are done with your day and want to turn in, there is a nighttime ritual that will also help you, and that is to decide what time you're going to go to bed and stick to a schedule. Planning sleep is critical to getting the most out of life, and I cannot stress the importance of a good night's sleep. Sleep is the number one longevity factor, because your body removes toxins from your brain when you sleep. You produce about twenty times the cerebrospinal fluid at night, and it is like you're washing the toxins out of your brain. This occurs when you are in deep sleep. This is the state of sleep that gives you healing and helps your body repair or regenerate your cells.

Sleep Deprivation

If you are sleeping less than six hours a day, you are sleep deprived, and I can tell you that you increase your chances of disease. A lack of sleep can wreak havoc on your body and predispose you to cardiovascular disease, impaired immunity, fading memory, hormone imbalances that can make you hungry all the time, and it can decrease the effectiveness to insulin release, which can make you vulnerable for prediabetes. Sleep deprivation not only makes you super tired and fatigued, it puts your body into a fight or flight state of stress. This fight or flight state increases your blood sugar, increases your LDL cholesterol and your heart rate, and shuts down the gut function, immune system function, and the serotonin levels as well as decreases your memory and body regeneration functions because your body is secreting stress hormones. Sleep deprivation causes your body to go through the same problems like if you were going through mental, physical, or chemical stress. It's almost like if you had experienced an auto accident. A decrease in gut health leads to depression, anxiety, and dementia. Take it from me, you need to sleep and sleep soundly for the best health and longevity. That means seven to eight hours of sleep per night, uninterrupted.

Helpful Ideas to Increase Sleep Hygiene

First of all, you should be relaxed at night for the last two hours of your day to put you in a good frame of mind. That means that watching the news is probably not a good idea because unfortunately, the news does not offer you feel-good stories before you sleep. Also using any electronic devices in the bedroom will cause you to alter your circadian rhythm, due to the artificial blue light. This blue light tricks your brain into thinking it is day time and keeps you awake. If you have an alarm clock, cover it so you don't see the blue glow. If you have to use a cellphone, turn on the blue light filter. Better yet, don't use your cellphone. Using heavy black out curtains helps you block out the light and dampen the noise. Try to not eat anything for three to four hours before bedtime so that you are not digesting food and gaining energy. If you have trouble relaxing before bedtime, you might need to have a cup of chamomile tea or a hot shower or bath to relax you so you can unwind. Prayer and meditation is great for the last hour while you are preparing for sleep, and journaling can help you unwind as well. You should be sleeping at least seven hours, so be mindful of the time. You can time yourself so you determine when you have to start getting ready for bed. The bedroom should be reserved for sleep only. This is not the place to exercise and do a lot of activities unrelated to sleep.

Sleeping Pills

I highly recommend you don't take sleeping pills as they cut your lifespan and don't give you a significant amount of extra sleep. The damaging effects of the pills are not warranted for the extra 15-30 minutes of sleep you might be gaining. When you take sleeping pills, you are not getting the REM sleep your body needs. Sleeping pills destroy your brain and can cause memory issues and lower your immunity. If you are having trouble sleeping, you need to reset your circadian rhythm. This can be done easily, but it takes consistency on your part. Go to bed at the same time every night, and wake up at the same time every day. When you wake up, stare into the blue sky (make sure this happens as soon as possible but at least within the first hour of waking up), as it reinforces that it is time to be awake.

Resetting the Circadian Rhythm

If you have tried the suggestions above, and you find that it is not working, and you find that you're awake and unable to sleep, then you may need to reset your circadian rhythm. In order to do this, you will need to undergo a temporary sleep deprivation schedule for twenty-one days to reset your circadian rhythm. It looks something like this: go to bed at 10-1030 and wake up at 4-430 for twenty-one days. When you wake up, look into the light, and it's ok to use your cell phone without the blue light filter at this point. The most important hours of the night to make sure you're asleep are between 11pm and 2am. In fact, the earlier you fall asleep before midnight, the better! Being able to sleep soundly and rest throughout the day will help reset your body's clock and help you experience the miracles of a good night's sleep. Proper sleep has wonderful benefits that include a true sense of wellbeing, increased body detoxification, improved cellular regeneration, improved memory, improved gut health, improved immunity, increased secretion of serotonin, normalization of blood pressure, blood sugar, and

LDL cholesterol. This, in turn, gives you an abundance of energy, joy, and vitality to get through your day so that you can accomplish all the things on your list. So remember, if you are having trouble sleeping or do not make it a priority, then decide to make that change because this is an easy step to really help you attain all your goals and dreams. Be good to your body and get some rest!

Chapter 8

Got Stress?

"It's really not the actual stress that kills us,
it is our reaction to it."
– Hans Selye

When you think of stress you may think of physical stress, mental stress, or biochemical stress. No matter what type of stress there is in the body, it causes your body to react. When you are healthy and are not stressed out, cortisol works in balance with DHEA (dehydrocpiandrosterone). Think of them as a seesaw. If you have the right amount of cortisol and the right amount of DHEA, the seesaw should be perfectly balanced, like kids that weigh the exact same amount. DHEA is your basic everything-is-going-pretty-well metabolic hormone. It gets secreted when things are going well. When stress overloads your body, the reaction is going to be increased cortisol levels (fight or flight reaction), which affects every other hormone in your body. And that is fine, it needs to go up to do that. The problem is when the body is under chronic stress, and cortisol stays elevated. This constant production of cortisol takes away from the adrenal gland's ability to actually produce DHEA. DHEA is a prohormone that is needed for almost 95% of all the hormones in your body. When you have issues with hormones that are caused by stress, you may go to your medical doctor and have them draw your blood to see these imbalances. Your doctor may recommend a shot, pill, patch, etc. And those might temporarily make you feel a little bit better, but it doesn't solve the underlying problem that the cortisol is up too high because of stress and the cortisol to DHEA ratio is completely out of whack.

Adrenal Fatigue

That means that the kid on the seesaw representing cortisol goes up, and the DHEA kid is closer to the ground. When DHEA goes down, these symptoms start to occur: you get fatigued, you get a decreased muscle mass, you lose bone density, you get depressed, your sex drive goes down, you're more susceptible to infections so you get sick and stay sick longer. As the cortisol level stays up and the adrenals are kicking out cortisol through fight or flight instead of allowing your nervous system and hormonal system to balance out the hormones, cortisol stays up there for a long time and then drops because it can't keep up with the production. It is like the seesaw arm that's up in the air breaks at the pivot point and it falls back down, and then everything gets even worse. You can call this adrenal exhaustion.

Adrenal Exhaustion

This is when you get significant issues with: chronic fatigue, depression, dizziness, lightheadedness, heart palpitations, anxiety, overall body aches, skin sensitivity that can cause diarrhea, vomiting, and abdominal pain that can get misdiagnosed as reflux or something else. You get hungry even if you just ate, causing weight gain, craving really salty food. You get clumsy and start to get confused. You can develop dark blue grey circles under the eyes, your period starts to get messed up, you get IBS symptoms, and you develop bladder issues where you have to go to the bathroom a lot more than usual!

Saliva Tests

How do you check to see if you have these stress hormones out of balance? Through saliva tests. Saliva tests gives you a picture of what's happening in your body all day long with the active levels of these hormones. There is a difference between saliva and blood tests. The saliva tests for active hormones and blood measures active and inactive hormones. Checking your hormone levels through the blood creates a problem because it is not necessarily accurate due to it checking for active as well as inactive hormone levels. Saliva tells you how you are doing now and how the hormones vary within a 24-hour period. If we check different saliva samples six times a day, then we can know exactly when the hormones begin to drop.

Solutions to Adrenal Fatigue and Adrenal Exhaustion

If we need to offer a solution due to an abnormal saliva test, we can determine exactly how much supplementation to give and at what exact time of day to recommend. You can vary the dose based on how you feel. We will only recommend all-natural remedies when necessary. They're chemically identical to what the body produces on its own, and it comes from a specific part of the wild yam plant. There's absolutely no side effects. The fact that they are sublingual makes them easily absorbed right into the blood stream. The drops are used to measure the exact amount that you may need. In fact, it gives you the elevation back to where the hormones should be so that you don't have to put chronic stress on the body while you rebuild the adrenal function with the capsule.

Adrenal Supplementation

Don't just take an arbitrary amount. If you decide to take an adrenal supplement, it's going to make you feel better, but we're actually trying to help you rebuild the gland that's worn out due to stress. If you don't have the blood chemistry functioning at a normal level while we rebuild the gland, does it make sense that we're really going to rebuild the gland? Everything else will stay out of balance. Remember the old seesaw example. If your cortisol levels are crashing in the middle of the day, that will affect your blood sugar, and that will affect your fat metabolism, your energy level, and everything else. The ratio is measuring the breaking down of the hormones vs. building up of the hormones. It's really a problem that affects blood sugar and how the cells utilize glucose, and if left out of balance, causes pre-diabetic issues or type 2 diabetes, that's where the problem arises. It can also affect the thyroid gland because thyroid stimulating hormones are produced in the pituitary, but measured in the hypothalamus. That's the same place where DHEA and cortisol are measured. You gain weight when you have a problem over time because you sacrifice normal blood sugar metabolism. Therefore, you are storing energy in fat cells, and when metabolism is out of balance, you keep craving food.

DHEA/cortisol ratio imbalance is the cause of the beginnings of many problems, especially feeling tired and fatigued. This should be checked on a regular basis. That's why we're so sick in this country! I can turn your life around by fixing this. The adrenal system is the most important hormone system in the body. There's no other system in the body that's responsible for producing over 95% of all the hormones. Without proper adrenal function, you will get sick and be susceptible to chronic debilitating illnesses, and that can affect your immune system. What happens when the immune system doesn't work? People get cancer, they get autoimmune diseases, degenerative aging diseases, blood sugar goes out of whack, you name it. This is a serious issue, and that is why I believe you need to look at it. When we fix the adrenal problem, these hormone levels will balance out almost immediately.

Screening Tests to Determine If Saliva Tests Are Needed

We do a couple tests before doing saliva tests to make sure you have a need. We check your blood pressure in a laying down position, then check it again while you're standing. The blood pressure should rise when you stand up by 10-15 points. If it stays the same or falls, then this can indicate adrenal problems. We also check the pupils of the eye to see how they react to light stimulus for 30 seconds. The pupils should get smaller when the light is shined in the eyes. If the pupils do not react to the light by getting smaller as to prevent light from entering the eye or they get smaller but are too tired to maintain that by getting bigger again that is a sign of weak adrenals. Have you gone out on a sunny day and felt you were being blinded by the light? I know people that have to wear sunglasses all the time because if they don't, they get a headache. These are signs of weak adrenals, and it may be advantageous to have a saliva test to check the levels. I recommend you do everything possible to see if your adrenals normalize on their own. Allow your body the chance to get healthy on its own, but if you have tried everything without a balance in your adrenals, and you are suffering from the symptoms mentioned above, then a saliva test could make all the difference in the world.

Physical Stress and the Nervous System

Sometimes your stress is physical in nature and it involves misalignments in the body. Thomas Edison said "the doctor of the future will give no medicine, but will interest his patients in the care of the human frame, in diet and prevention of disease." When functioning as a chiropractor, my main job is to make sure that your nervous system is free and clear of any irritation on the delicate nerves that are exiting the spine. This allows you to feel great and be super productive. Your brain controls every cell, every tissue, and every organ in your entire body. When all is well, you function normally and your body works like a machine. There is no strain or any problems when there is normal nervous system function. That is what we want. However, unfortunately, life happens, and we have physical stress placed in our bodies, and that can cause irritation on the nerves as they exit the spine. We call this misaligned bones or subluxations.

If you have pressure or irritation on your nerves, how well do you think you're going to work? Not very well. If those are the nerves in the upper neck that control blood flow to the head and neck, then how well are those areas going to work? Not very well. You can have nerve pressure and irritations going on in your body and not even know it because only about 18 percent of the nerve fibers transmit pain signals. When you have pressure on the nerves in your body, the functions go down whether you are aware of it or not. Over time, your body begins to have difficulty functioning properly. There is a lack of ease, and you start to create a state of dis-ease in your body. Left uncorrected, that lack of ease can eventually turn into a disease which would be defined as abnormal cells and tissues that we can see on x-rays or other tests. This happens all the time. I can tell you that there are many people running around in this world with subluxations, malfunction, and diseases and they don't even know about it. When people have subluxations, this condition decreases the functions in the affected parts by 60 percent, leaving them with about 40 percent function. Left uncorrected over more time, you eventually get symptoms of one sort or another. This is when most of my patients come and see me and what they want is for their symptoms to go away. What would you rather have disappear? The symptom or the cause of the problem? If you don't fix the root of the problem but only are concerned with eliminating the symptom, then the problem will continue to worsen over time and the symptoms will reappear because the problem was there all along. Make sure to decide on what you want in the long run so that you can live healthily and have lasting, permanent results. Make sure to see a chiropractor that is in alignment with your core values and can offer you what you want.

What to Expect in a Chiropractic Office on the First Visit

When I see a new patient, I always consult with them first to see if their complaints are a chiropractic problem that I can fix, and if so, I check them for these subluxations to see if their problems are physical. If so, then I check to see how bad it is and if there are any complicating factors involved that would delay the process. Once I determine if it is a chiropractic problem that I can most likely help, we get started by doing an examination and x-rays if necessary.

Keeping the Communication Lines Open

What we want to do is educate you on your case so that you can make all the right decisions based on what your goals are. If you can't perform your activities of daily life, then treatment has to be geared toward fixing you so that you can do what you desire. There is nothing worse in this world than not being able to do what you love. You may want to ride your horse with your girlfriends or go golfing or run a marathon. I believe you should do whatever it is that your heart desires.

Remember the brain controls every part of your body. Anything that interferes with the signals from the brain to different parts of the body is bad. Anything that takes the interference off the nervous system and allows it to function properly again is good. That is what chiropractic is all about. Chiropractic allows the body to heal itself by taking the pressure off the nervous system, and that is a good thing. When given the opportunity to function well, the body will heal.

Your Body's Foundation

It is important to make sure that your structure is balanced from your feet on up to your head. I have seen so many problems that start due to improper balance in the feet, and they translate all the way up the spine. There could be five things wrong with you. If that is the case, then you need to fix all five things in order to resolve the problem so it doesn't come back. When we are treating the spine and we find the bones are not aligned properly, then it usually involves more than just putting the bones back into the proper alignment. You have to realize that joints that are soft and supple function well and stay healthy. When you have a misaligned bone, it not only irritates a nerve, but it can cause a muscle spasm that holds the joint out of alignment. That, in turn, causes ligaments to be over stretched in an awkward position, and this causes lack of normal joint motions that fixate the joint and don't allow the fluid motion to occur. Maybe the joint is restricted in one way or moves in an uneven way, and this can eventually put uneven pressure on the joint and cause degeneration in the disc and spine. Whatever the issues are, it must be determined that if full correction is going to occur, you need the pressure and irritation to be removed from the nerve, but then you need to make sure the muscles are balanced so that the muscles do not pull you off again. The ligaments need to be rehabilitated so the joint is not lax and unstable, and the proper motion needs to be restored in all directions, and then the degeneration that has begun needs to be stopped. This is what insures perfect and proper correction so that the problem does not return, and you do not have predisposing factors that would cause future problems. This is accomplished by looking at all the factors that cause these subluxations – which are many times posturally related – in addition to any injuries sustained.

Fixing Your Posture

You must check for imbalances in the body and fix them so that they do not become permanent issues. When your body has a slumped posture, for instance, you can be treated with the best intentions but your problem will not fully go away if the postural changes are not addressed. This, in turn, will zap your energy.

Remember the stretch I gave you that had you taking a short break to look up, open the chest, and squeeze your shoulder blades together? That stretch is going to help you a lot not only in gaining energy, but in fixing your posture. You will look better, too. You have to stretch your chest muscles and strengthen your upper back for fifteen to twenty seconds every fifteen to twenty minutes. If you have a forward head posture (which is common), then that will need to be addressed as well, otherwise you will never fully resolve your issues. If you sit all day at a desk, then you're also going to have problems and imbalances in the lower back region and pelvis, which will need to be addressed differently. I bet you have tight hamstring muscles and hip flexor muscles from sitting so long, and weak glutes and abs. Remember you don't get buns of steel from sitting on them. **Download the Free companion PDF to this book at NoMoreFatigueextras.com.**

Rehabilitation of Joints

I find that when you really want to fix the problem in the fastest way, you first need to mobilize the spine and joints. Once there is some fluidity in the joints, you can then stretch them, and then you strengthen and stabilize the surrounding areas. You don't want to start strengthening the muscles around the joints in the wrong position and posture because that defeats the purpose. Mobilize first, stretch second, and strengthen last.

Pressure Point Therapy

One of the things I enjoy teaching to the employees of my corporate clients is pressure point therapy. This helps them feel more energized, feel less pain and tightness, and maintain better posture. Don't worry, you won't be sweating up a storm. Pressure point therapy helps relieve blocked energy coming from nerve interference. It helps improve flexibility, increase range of motion, blood flow, and energy, and decrease muscle spasms, stress, and pain. It is easy to perform and helps immediately in some cases. First you have to locate the point using your thumbs, and what you're looking for is a hard painful nodule in the meaty part of the muscles, then you want to hold PRESSURE equal to 2-5 times the pressure that would be comfortable on your eye (NO More). Remember this is not revenge time! You want to count to twelve, or leave on until it melts it away. You then repeat on the opposite side because anything done to the left, you should do to the right. But really concentrate treating the painful spots. You then move to next lower point. Always work from highest point to lowest moving from central to peripheral. Then repeat on the tender spots. Only have your partner work on you for about three to five minutes so they are willing to do this again and again in the future. It would be great if you could do this several times a week. When this energy is released, you will feel better and more energized.

This, of course, is the physical part of what we call the triad. The triad is an equilateral triangle with three equal parts that represent the physical or structural part of health, the mental or emotional part of health, and the biochemical part of health. All three areas have to be healthy for you to be healthy. If you have a physical problem, then you require a physical solution; if you have a mental/emotional problem, then you require a mental solution; and if you have a biochemical imbalance, then you will require a biochemical solution. The good news is that if you improve any one area of this triangle, then the others will be positively affected as well. I hope you are able to see and understand just how detrimental the effects of stress can be on the body both physically, chemically as well as mentally, and I hope you will decide to minimize the effects as much as possible so that you can feel great and be super productive in everything you do.

Q&A of Energy Enhancements with Chiropractic

How does manual cracking differ from computer guided chiropractic adjustments?

Before seeking chiropractic care, always ask any questions you may have regarding the process. Some of the questions or comments that come up are as follows. You're scared and don't want to have your neck cracked. I get it. It can be concerning if you're finding it difficult to relax. If you're not completely relaxed, it's going to hurt. There is no actual cracking of the actual bones with chiropractic care, but rather the release of gaseous pressure built up into the joints when they get stiff and stuck together and are not moving properly. In my office, and some other offices around the world, there is a new computer guided chiropractic evaluation and treatment instrument that is gentle and does not require any twisting and turning and snapping or cracking of the neck or spine. We analyze the spine using the instrument and then choose the bones we want to adjust, adjust them, and reanalyze the spine to see how the adjustment worked. It gives us real time information so that we can decide when to adjust and when not to adjust. The instrument is gentle and very precise and shuts off automatically so that you don't get under adjusted or over adjusted. You get exactly what you need for that day.

Can you get addicted?

Because there are no addicting chemicals involved, chiropractic is not addictive. However, when you feel so good and you like the new flexibility, mobility and decreased pain, you will want more.

Once you go for chiropractic care, do you always have to go?

That's not the case. In my office, we have different kinds of care – relief care, corrective care, and maintenance care. Our patients decide what kind of care they want, and we support them in their decision. Relief care is the care necessary to feel better, but not actually totally fix the underlying root of the problem. Corrective care is the care necessary to feel better and fix the underlying root of the problem so it doesn't come back. Maintenance care is the care some people choose once they are better so they can stay better. The bottom line is that there is a beginning, middle, and end to care, and you get to choose what kind of care you want. I have found many people that feel so good that they keep on coming for maintenance care, but that is up to them.

One of my patients made a comment that she would really like her husband to be a patient too, because he has problems but he doesn't believe in chiropractic. I responded that chiropractic is not a religion, so it will work even though you don't believe as long as his problem is a chiropractic one that can be fixed. Maybe someone you know has tried chiropractic in the past and had a bad experience, and now they don't ever want to see a chiropractor. I can tell you that there are good and bad chiropractors just like there are good and bad restaurants, good and bad plumbers, good and bad teachers, and the list goes on and on. There are good and bad people in any profession and I'm going to say we're one of the good ones and let me tell you why. I always do a thorough consultation with you to see if you even qualify to receive services, and that is followed by a thorough examination to determine just how bad you really are and if there are any complicating factors that could affect the outcome. Then I determine what the treatment, if any, needs to be for your individual case. I go over that before we start any care whatsoever so that you can decide what you want to do. You have to decide how bad the problem is and if it is ruining your life and if you want to get rid of it so you can be happy and healthy again so that you can do all the things you want to do. You may want that or not.

I have found that some people just don't care to fix their problems because it hasn't yet ruined their lives. That's completely up to them. You are the one that has to be interested in fixing your problems, not me. It doesn't do me any good to want to help you if you don't want the help. I want to help you if you want to be helped, otherwise it doesn't work because you won't do all the things you really need to do to get the best results. I want to help you get well and be able to do all those things you want to do so you can be happy and have your dreams come true. But the choice has to come from you first.

I have a patient in my office who's in his late 70s, and he is one that has been coming to me for many years. He is feeling great and wants to continue with his care on a maintenance basis. He made the decision on his own and he sees the value of receiving care and feels terrific with care. He realizes he is only getting older, and since he feels so good and is able to do all the things he wants to do, he wants to keep doing it. It's funny, this gentleman owns many apartments in Los Angeles and still manages them all himself. He does some of the handy work himself and wants to continue to be active. He sees the value of keeping his spine in alignment and keeping his joints soft and supple so that he can stop any further degeneration in his joints, but most of all keep his energy levels up to tackle the day full speed ahead.

Chapter 9

Attitude, Feelings, and Law of Resonance

Remember the triangle, the triad that encompasses your health and wellbeing as it relates to your energy and vitality? One side of the triangle is the structural component. Another side is the biochemical component. The third side is the mental, emotional part. Each side is equally important and represents one third of your health picture.

Your emotions are mirroring your life. What I mean by that is, if you're a negative person, then you're going to face some challenges, because you'll be vibrating at a frequency that will be bringing into your reality those things that vibrate at the same level. This is a law of the universe, and whether you believe in it or not, it is happening. The law is called the Law of Resonance. Have you ever been so happy that everything in your life was going great and it all flowed effortlessly? You were full of energy and felt like you were on cloud nine and could get so much done easily. Or maybe you're on the other end where everything is hard and you feel like there is no way you can get it all done, you're frustrated and exhausted and can't even imagine getting through the day. You dread waking up and dread going to work and your energy levels are nil. When you are vibrating at a higher vibration, you are attracting more health and energy into your life.

There are many ways to vibrate higher, but first, figure out where you are right now. As you read these words, I want you to notice how you're feeling right now. Are you happy, are you sad, are you anxious, overwhelmed, or bored? Try to notice what you're feeling. While noticing what emotions come up, breathe deeply and don't judge them. Just notice. Be mindful of what you are noticing as you go through your day and don't try to change it for now but just notice it.

In order to make the necessary changes in life, first you have to notice where you are right now. You might want to write down your predominant feelings so that you know where you are. After doing this, you can begin to see what vibrations you're coming from. As you become more aware, I want you to take inventory of what makes you happy and inspires you and gives you energy, and what makes you sad or sucks the life out of you. Without making any changes yet, just keep noticing so that you can begin to see the patterns in your life.

Many talk about self-love, but what does that really mean to you? Does it mean that you love yourself, or does it mean that you take better care of yourself, or does it mean that you support yourself in your dreams or aspirations? When I think of self-love, I think of it as my body is my temple and I want to treat it well on all three levels of the triad. I want to physically take good care of myself and do whatever it takes to be healthy and well, and mentally take care of myself so that I'm not so critical and judgmental about myself. I want to biochemically take care of myself so that I expose my body to things that are good in nature and will help me achieve better health and vitality. And when exposed to those things in life that we cannot avoid, I want to be able to do what I can to minimize any damaging effects.

When you have a puppy or small child, how do you treat them? Most people would say they nurture them and give them all the things they need which would include healthy food, water, and love, to name a few. We don't tend to yell at the puppy or small child because we know they are young and helpless and need to be nurtured. Unfortunately, we do not always give ourselves the same treatment. I like to think of my inner child as a baby that needs to be loved and nurtured so that I can treat her right and love her so that she can grow like a flower. We don't always realize how critical we can be of ourselves, or how critical we are of others when we get on the critical vibration.

How do you talk to yourself? Do you talk to yourself like a baby that's just learning how to walk or talk? Do you criticize yourself consciously or even unconsciously? I'm here to say that we just need to be mindful of how we treat ourselves and others because that sets the vibration that we will be on. It's like a thermostat that you set in your house. Once you set it, it kicks in to either heat up or cool down the house or keep you where you're at. If you're not happy with the temperature, you just reset it and go from there. Unfortunately, it is not that easy to change the thermostats of your feelings without mindfully making those changes.

If you don't change the thermostat, then when it gets cooler or hotter in our home, it automatically changes based on where you set the thermostat. When you want to make changes in our lives and be happier mentally, you can try to do that and you can succeed temporarily, but that darn thermostat will bring you back down to where you were before. So in order to make the necessary long term changes at a higher level, you need to be intentional and mindful of where you are and where you want to be.

Vibrate Higher

How do you get to a place where you're vibrating on a higher level? You practice. One of the most positive and higher levels you can vibrate at is that of love. When you feel love, notice what it feels like, notice the vibration. Gratitude is also a positive vibration you want to strive to be in as much as possible. To reach a vibration of gratitude, write down what you're grateful for in your life each and every morning. Feel gratitude for at least five minutes, and raise your vibration. Even express gratitude on your way to the bathroom. Also think about what you are proud of about yourself. It's like treating yourself as a small child that has just taken her first step. Maybe you can feel proud of yourself for taking the five minutes today and feeling gratitude for being alive, maybe you're grateful for having the eyes to see the beauty in the day or the legs to go out for a run or anything at all that you feel grateful for. Just feel that gratitude inside of you!

As you practice this, you slowly start to raise your own thermostat so that life doesn't keep bringing you down. If you do this on a hit or miss basis, it will not be enough to raise your thermostat. Make the simple decision to make this one change, and I can tell you that you will be so much better off as a result.

Thoughts are things and they all have a certain vibration. If you're negative, then that will be the vibration of your life, and you will attract more negative things in your life that are at the same vibration. Personally, I do not watch the news because it is so negative. I feel bad when I do, so I decided not to watch it anymore. I try to keep my world as positive as possible because I understand how important it is to my life and everything I do. I am human and sometimes things cause me to get angry or sad or experience pain, but because I am mindful, I notice it and get into gratitude again or think of my grandchildren who I love so much and that always brings me back. It is not easy, but it is achievable. You need to get in the habit of being in gratitude. That is easy and it will raise your vibration.

If you are unwilling to raise yourself up and vibrate at higher levels, you just won't do it, and you will be living the life that corresponds to the thermostat you set in your past. If you aren't happy with your current situation, then you need to make a change. Nothing changes on its own, you need to intentionally decide where you are now and where you want to be. Think about what you want in in life. Think about what you don't want any longer. This is your life and you get to design it however you want. Don't wait until it's too late and you're on your deathbed full of regret. Decide to do something now. Someone once told me that in life, we don't get what we deserve, we get what we believe we deserve. I agree with that statement completely and have seen that in my own life and in the many lives I have touched over the years. I practice affirmations and visualizations and yes I have a vision board in my bathroom that I look at every day when I'm brushing my teeth and getting ready in the morning and getting ready for bed in the evening. I have been saying affirmations for over 30 years daily, and I am acutely aware of the "I am" affirmation and I believe it is the most powerful of all the affirmations. What that means is when you say "I am sick all the time" or "I am tired" or whatever you say after the "I am," that sets your vibration.

As a doctor, I treat many people with all different kinds of issues, and when they complain to me about how horrible they feel sometimes, they are putting so much emotion into that feeling that it sets their vibration. As part of my treatment, when I have patients who are frequently emotionalizing how horrible their life is, I have them write down their complaints so I know what to address. Then no matter how they feel, I have them affirm positive statements such as: I am well, I am perfect in every way, I am so healthy and so energized. Doing this shifts their vibration and allows my treatments to work better, and quite frankly it helps them whether they get treatment or not. If they just can't bring themselves to say it because it feels like a lie that they cannot overcome, then I have them affirm "every day in every way, I am getting better and better." The bottom line is that sometimes you have to fake it to make it. You have to be an actor. I promise you it gets easier to do it and the feelings and vibrations you are at when you are affirming "I am well" is so much better than saying "why can't I get well," "why am I so messed up," or "I can never have enough energy."

I challenge you to practice positive affirmations for twenty-one days and see how your life changes. Problems with your thoughts and feelings rank up there with the physical or biochemical issues you may be experiencing. It won't hurt you to try, so do yourself a favor and either decide to do this wholeheartedly or decide to give it your best effort. Whatever you do, don't say the words "I am well" while feeling, "No, I'm not!" Once you've been doing this for a while, notice what happens in your life. Notice the changes. When we have goals of achieving whatever it is we want to in life, like wanting more energy, or a promotion at work, or more money, etc., you should ask yourself a few questions like:

- If I got that, would that make me happy?
- Does it align with my values in life?
- Does it cause me to grow in a good way?
- Does this help others as well as myself?

When you answer yes to these questions, you know you're on the right track. It will be sustainable because it will not only be good for you personally, but it aligns with the greater good of others.

My final words on this is for you to do your best in every situation you are faced with. If you fall short, no worries. Just take a few deep breaths. Don't play the blame or shame game because it is not useful. Try putting a Post-it note up on the wall or on your computer with the words "I am _____" fill in the blank with a word or words that positively inspire you. When you feel any doubt, remember to keep repeating over and over whatever affirmation makes the biggest change in you. "I am capable," "I am more than enough," or "I rock!" As you get better at this, you will continue to grow and achieve greater benefits. Always be mindful of where you are so you can course-correct if necessary and live in gratitude. When you live in gratitude, you will be happier, smile more, be more relaxed, and be pleasant to be around. Remember you get what you expect, so expect the best! Your attitude will determine your success or failure. Henry Ford said, "Whether you think you can or think you can't – you're right."

Breathing Techniques

In true moments of sadness, you need to allow yourself to feel those feelings and then move on when you're ready. Don't stay there. Take three to six deep breaths and focus. Breathe in love and breathe out sadness. Breathe in gratitude and breathe out fear. When you feel you have experienced enough sadness and want to move on but can't, then remember to get back into gratitude and love. Positivity and gratitude will make all the difference in the world, and will help you vibrate at higher frequencies which allow you experience things you never dreamed possible.

It is very difficult to be tired when you are feeling so grateful for your life and vibrating at those higher frequencies.

Chapter 10

How Does Exercise Increase Your Energy Levels?

I n order to keep the energy in your body flowing you need to move your body. When you move your body you feel alive. The more you move the more energy you feel. Your cells actually vibrate at a higher level. If you are not moving your body you get rigid and your energy goes down because your cells are vibrating at a lower frequency. The ultimate state of lack of movement is 6 feet under. Exercise is one of the easiest ways to gain energy. There are many ways to accomplish this. I recommend you do what you love to do so that it doesn't even feel like exercising. Just move your body and keep moving your body every day. Maybe that's a walk outside, maybe walking your dog, dancing, skiing, or taking a swim. There's so much to choose from. Breathe in deeply and rhythmically as you move. If you don't know what to do yet, you should consider a combination of aerobic and anaerobic types of exercise.

Aerobic Exercise

When I think of aerobic exercise, I think of dancing, power walking or running, and it involves rhythmic movement without stopping. If you haven't exercised for a while, think about taking it super slow and just start by walking. Walk for five to ten minutes, then see how you're doing. If you don't have any physical issues, then I recommend walking for longer, but check with your doctor first and make sure it is safe for you. A good rule of thumb is to exercise twenty to thirty minutes a day, but remember if you have not done it for a while or have never done it, then start slow.

When you exercise, make sure you're not holding your breath. For instance, if you're walking, breathe with your steps (breathe in for four counts and breathe out for four counts) to your own rhythm. This will help you oxygenate your body. Your muscles need oxygen and nutrients so they can work well. Oxygen is carried by your blood to feed your muscles. Aerobic exercise carries lots of oxygen to your muscles, and it can be sustained for greater periods of time without feeling out of breath. The benefit is not only feeling energized, but also gaining better cardiovascular health and burning fat, as well as improving your moods.

I also think performing aerobic exercise is great for energy because of the increase in maximal oxygen uptake, or VO2 max. While doing aerobic exercise, if you're fit, then you will have a slower heart rate, slower breathing rate, and less muscle fatigue and ton of energy as compared to if you were out of shape. Don't get discouraged if you can't do that much at first. With practice and patience, you will improve. Consistency is the key, and even if you don't feel like it, get out and move your body and breathe deeply. You will find yourself able to do more and more over time, and you will be setting yourself up for stress reduction, increased energy and vitality, and overall health and wellbeing.

Anaerobic Exercise

When you perform anaerobic exercises like lifting weights, you can lose breath more rapidly. These exercises do not distribute oxygen in the same way as aerobic exercises. It is mainly when you have short bursts of exercise at higher intensities like sprinting or weightlifting. You may perform a set of ten to twelve reps at a time and then rest.

Anaerobic exercise increases your metabolic rate with greater intensity than aerobic exercise. When you run, for instance, your metabolic rate can go up for a couple hours after you stop, but when you lift weights, your metabolic rate can go up and stay up for several days. Your basal metabolic rate is the amount of energy per unit of time that keeps your body functioning at rest. A high basal metabolic rate gives you more energy and allows you to do more than if it were too low. As we age, we lose about 2 percent of our basal metabolic rate for every ten years starting at around twenty. If you have more muscle mass, then you should have a higher basal metabolic rate than someone that has less muscle and more fat.

When you're lifting weights, start slowly and increase the repetitions and weight over time. I promise you that you will get stronger. Make sure you're capable of doing it by talking with your doctor first. There may come a time when you can no longer lift heavier weight safely and without injuries, so you may want to increase the repetitions or even the times per week that you lift. Getting a personal trainer to help you is always a plus, as they can make sure you are using proper form and can help you make realistic goals so that you can improve without injuries.

Metabolic Rate

In general, women have lower basal metabolic rates than men. How do you increase it? You need to work out more and gain muscle tissue. As you work out, you start to get fitter and fitter, and over time, you will need to do more and more. Doing the same workout routine over and over is fine at first, but then you need to change it. You need to challenge yourself more in order to keep receiving positive gains and increasing your muscle mass and cellular engines.

Remember when we talked about how the mitochondria in your cells were responsible for energy production and how the more mitochondria you have and/or the size of the mitochondria is important if you are trying to increase your energy levels? Think of it this way. If you have too few mitochondria or they are small, delicate little guys, then your energy levels will be less than what you may desire. In order to get your mitochondria to grow in size and number, you need to place a demand on them similar to what exercise does on your muscle cells. If you don't move and breathe and demand more of yourself every day, then you won't be needing more mitochondria, bigger mitochondria. Any type of exercise will help you develop and grow your cellular engines.

***

If you are not already fit, any type of exercise will be beneficial for you whether it is aerobic or anaerobic types of exercise. Just start moving your body. If you are trying to increase muscle mass in order to increase your metabolic rate, then I would recommend lifting weights so that you can build greater muscle mass and that in turn will help you to increase your energy.

A fit person, however, will need to do both aerobic and anaerobic types of exercise to continue to grow their cellular engines. Imagine if you do grow the numbers and the size of your mitochondria. You can double, triple, or even quadruple your energy. It only takes intention to do a little more than what you did before. Maybe what increases is the time you take to exercise, or the demands during exercise, or both. Either way, you build your cellular engines and enjoy the benefits of more and more energy than you have today.

And don't forget to breathe deeply while exercising, as that increases your metabolic fire, and for those of you wanting to gain energy and even lose a couple of pounds, this is important. Think of your metabolic fire as a wildfire. If you live in California like me, we get concerned when we have Santa Ana winds due to the possibility of wildfires. When we do have these wildfires, the winds just fuel them and they rage out of control. If your metabolic fire is that of a candle instead of a wildfire, all you have to do is have a small breeze and it goes out. The way this relates to energy is that in order to have sustained energy with exercise, you need to have a strong metabolic fire burning inside of you. This keeps you energized and going for a long time. You don't want to have a weak small candle inside you that goes out at the first sign of a breeze. The same goes for eating for energy. If you have a raging fire inside, you can eat more food and sometimes even eat the wrong kinds of foods, and it won't really affect you too much because the fire inside you will burn it up easily.

But if your fire has gone out, and you only have smoldering coals left, you can't utilize the food you eat for energy, so it just sits there and turns into fat, making you more tired.

Posture Correction and Stretching

When we sit at a desk for instance and work on a computer all day, certain bad postures develop and, if not checked, can cause bigger problems later. The upper body goes into a slouching type of posture with a forward head and the lower part of your body develops an imbalance due to sitting too long. Besides not being very attractive, this kind of posture can have far reaching effects on our energy as well as the tension we feel in our neck, shoulders and back. Slumped posture can also have a detrimental effect on lung capacity. It is important to take a break periodically and move your body, and at the very least, do a stretch as described before where you look up as far back as possible, opening your chest and holding for fifteen to twenty seconds. It's even better when you can stand up and do it standing so your lower back gets a chance to rest and change its posture. I recommend you stand up and look up and back while opening your chest and taking three deep breaths with your palms facing forward as you squeeze your shoulder blades together. Always add a yawn if you can, too, as that can help stop the negative effects of the stress that you may be experiencing or other feelings of negativity. Then before you sit down, stretch to the side raising one arm up, and reach for the sky and over while the other arm touches the side of your thigh and below your knee. Repeat this stretch on the other side. And then place your hands on your hips and lean backwards like you're doing a back bend, and feel the stretch in your hips. You want to hold all the different positions for fifteen to twenty seconds each side, and don't forget to breathe.

If you can't do them all, alternate different stretches to affect the different parts of your body that get tight while sitting. Be mindful of what's happening to you and the tension you feel in your body as you slowly stretch. By slowly I mean like you can hardly see movement happening. This allows any painful areas to relax while you're doing it. Give your brain a chance to notice the tension and send down a signal to that muscle to allow for a relaxation response. While you do this, be careful not to rush the movements as you might pull something and make it worse.

The benefits of stretching last about an hour, so if you're stretching once or twice a day, while better than nothing, it is not enough. You need to stretch more often. If you stretch every twenty minutes, that is three times per hour, and you will be making a huge difference in your recovery rate and stretching ability. If you only stretch once per hour that's great, but you won't be getting all the results you truly want.

It's important for your posture to move and breathe and exercise, this is something you can do while working that helps you get through the day easier when a project is due and you're glued to your desk. You want to pay particular attention to your chest, upper trapezius muscles, lower back, hip flexors, and hamstrings. These are the muscles that are susceptible to shortening when sitting at a desk doing computer work or during other daily activities. When stretching any muscle that is tight, just think of the action of the muscle and do the opposite to stretch it. For example, you can stretch your hamstrings easily by putting your foot on the chair and lowering your body towards your knee, holding the stretch on each side for fifteen to thirty seconds. The trapezius muscles can be stretched by bending your neck sideways like you are trying to have your ear reach your shoulder while anchoring your opposite shoulder down.

For balance, stretch in both directions. This should not hurt, but you should feel a stretch. If there is pain, stop immediately. Avoid trying to strengthen tight muscles because doing so may cause more of an imbalance in your body. Other muscles tend to get weak due to being over-stretched. Those muscles should be strengthened. You may feel pain or tightness in some muscles no matter what. If simple stretching does not help, this indicates that there is a problem that you should have looked at by a professional. For example, the quadriceps or front of the thighs tend to be over stretched due to sitting for long periods of time. These muscles should stretch easily when stretched. However, if it hurts to stretch those, that can indicate a pelvic distortion due to tight quadriceps or even tight hip flexor muscles which are very common, and cause pelvic imbalances that need to be corrected. Either way, you should be able to identify what is tight and gently stretch it, and over time, you will have a better postural balance.

A visit to your chiropractor or physical therapist can also identify muscle imbalances if you cannot figure out the root cause or why stretching or exercising isn't helping. The main point you should remember is don't sit too long, take breaks, stretch tight muscles, and strengthen weak muscles.

Always consult your physician before beginning any exercise program. If you experience any pain or difficulty with these exercises, stop, and consult your healthcare provider.

Chapter 11

Plan Your Life and Manage Your Time

"Doing something that is productive is a great
way to alleviate stress. Get your mind doing
something that is productive."
– Ziggy Marley

Y ou might say that you don't have enough time to get everything done, but we all have twenty-four hours a day. What we do with that time to make it productive is another matter altogether. If you are falling short, then let me recommend a few things I have been able to do over the years. Focus is key to getting anything done, and you must prioritize what you want to accomplish this week, this month, and this very day. It only takes some time to plan and I'm sure you've heard the saying if you fail to plan, then you plan to fail. Make no mistake about it, everything you do in life and do well takes planning. Planning increases the focus of your activities and action steps in completing tasks and projects. I like to plan on Sunday nights. For an hour, I plan the upcoming week and check the calendar for any upcoming tasks and projects. I look at my deadlines and determine what needs to be done and make a plan. If it's important and urgent, then I set the time to get it done. If it is too big of a project to complete in one sitting, then I may allow a few hours per day to do part of it until it is done. I make note of the deadline and get it in my calendar. Since I don't have lots of free time in between working with clients, I make sure to give myself a bit of extra time in order to accommodate an emergency. Do this so your projects don't become emergencies.

I write all my activities and appointments for the whole week in a calendar and every night I look at what I need to get done the very next day, and prioritize what gets done first and how much time I need and when I will be getting it done. If I don't do it the night before, I find myself wasting time the next morning to figure it out. Besides, I sleep better when I know I have a plan to tackle my next day.

I also schedule time to look at emails and my inbox, but I try not to spend too much time on this, as I've found this is a big time waster. More on that later. When I get ready to sit down and work, I like to make sure my desk is not full of piles of work everywhere and super cluttered because my brain does not work well when there are piles of unfinished work all around me. Granted that happens sometimes, but I find myself so much less productive. There's a name for people who have stacks of work all over their desks. Stackers! Don't be a stacker! All that unfinished work leads to mental stress and mental stress causes your productivity to suffer. It's like having too many thoughts in your mind about all the things you have to do. Get it out of your head and put it down on paper and get organized.

One of my favorite books on time management is David Allen's *Getting Things Done*. I liked it so much after reading the book that I also got it on audio, so that I could make sure I was keeping all my stuff under control. Believe me, I used to be a stacker, and it was very stressful for me. My brain didn't work well with clutter all around me. Now I keep my very large desk organized, and get a bit bothered when my staff thinks they can use it to organize their work. I do not want anyone putting anything on my desk, least of all more work.

When it comes to emails, I like to keep my "inbox" separate as that can be a daunting thing to look at. When I get to my scheduled time to look at my "inbox," I ask myself several questions. "Does this need to be done?" "If so, does it need to be done now, or can I schedule it for later?" If it needs to be done, I ask, "how long will it take me to do it?" If it will take me less than one to two minutes, I like to do it right then and there, so I don't have to write it down and calendar it. If it takes longer than two minutes, I ask myself, "do I have to do it, or can I delegate it to someone else?" If I don't have to do it, then I will place it in someone else's inbox. If I'm the only one that can do it and it takes longer than two minutes to do, then I write it down on my to-do list and indicate where I can find the information to do it. Some things that come across my desk don't have actionable steps, and I may choose to file it away. And some things I just throw in the trash. Here is how I sort my "inbox" into other boxes:

- To do now or to do later
- Delegate to someone else
- To pay
- To read
- To file
- To throw it away in the trash, which is my favorite and easiest way to get things off my plate

In fact, I always have my trash can ready next to me when I open mail and sort through my inbox. I don't want to have to make it difficult for me to throw it away. Decide if it will be the end of the world or hurt you in any way if you throw it away. Maybe you could find the information again even faster if you Google it rather than sorting through papers.

In order to save time, I also try to stick to a rule I have of looking and touching things only once, if possible. If I don't stick it in the appropriate box, then when I touch it again later, I have to go through deciding what I have to do again and again every time I come across it. That is a big waste of time and leads to more stress. So try to touch it only once and put it where you can deal with it later. That is how I deal with all the papers that come across my desk and, for the most, part I have solved that problem.

Another time waster is emails. I don't know about you, but I get hundreds of emails every day and it is difficult to deal with sometimes. But the worst is when you are emailing someone and going back and forth and the subject line doesn't change or there is no subject line. That drives me crazy. I don't know how many times I have spent way too much time trying to look for an email with information that I needed because there was either a back and forth conversation that didn't have a subject line, or the conversation topic changed and the subject line didn't change. Subject lines should be as specific as possible so you can quickly find the email you want to find without wasting too much time opening a bunch of emails. My staff knows that is what I need, and if someone that I am dealing with sends me an email that I will need to reference later, then I change the subject line and send my reply. Just like junk mail that comes in the mail, there is junk mail that comes to your email, and you should quickly identify and delete as soon as possible or just don't bother opening up. Periodically, I do a major dump of old emails to clean out my files, as that is mental clutter for me too. I keep what I absolutely need, and I ask myself would it kill me to throw this away. If the answer is no, then it's gone.

When you can organize your schedule, work, and emails this way, your energy will go up as will your productivity and you will feel in control of your life instead of a victim to everything and everybody that is pulling you in all different directions. If you are a stacker, do yourself a favor and get rid of all those piles of incomplete activities you have all around you and start feeling better today. You'll be amazed at how that simple act of organization will make you feel empowered and energized.

Lastly, there is Facebook, and I only mention it because I have to limit my access to it because it will consume an amazing amount of time. Don't get me wrong, I love seeing what my friends and family are up to and all those cute pictures of our fur babies and people wishing each other happy birthday. But when I have deadlines, I do not get on Facebook at all. In fact, I turn off notifications from my phone entirely while working on my projects, otherwise those distractions can eat up my entire day and the only time I have to work on paperwork and projects is when I am not actually treating patients and or coaching clients. My advice to you is to plan what you're going to do, when you're going to do it, how long you're going to do it, and stick to that plan as best you can. Otherwise, things just won't get done because something always comes up that might be easier or more enjoyable to do.

Plan Your Life and Get Things Done

Don't live in crisis mode getting things done at the last minute because that leads to lots of stress, and as you now know, stress affects your hormones and every part of your life in a negative way. When you meet your deadlines and get things done, you are essentially taking care of yourself and making time to have fun and enjoy family and friends. I can tell you back before I learned these methods of planning my life, when I was in school, all I did was study. I had no time for anything else. My family would go on vacations and I couldn't go because I was studying all the time. I remember after I graduated and got married and had my daughter, it was still hard to carve out time to do it all. I missed so many family gatherings while I was doing well in practice and studying for my orthopedic board. My parents planned a wonderful vacation for the whole family back when my daughter was around four. My ex-husband and daughter got to go to Lake Shasta and spend a week there on a house boat with my whole family and all the cousins. I didn't get to go because I didn't know back then how to manage my time properly. I heard it was a great time and I missed it, and it was a sad time for me. Now I know how to plan my life and organize it so I can have fun, too. Don't do what I did back then.

I can't stress enough that you have to plan and organize your life so that you can get it all in there, including fun times with family and friends. I plan out my time so that I can have it all. I plan time for activities to strengthen my relationships with my family and friends doing those things I love to do, and that brings them joy, too. I plan time to work on my health and get my exercise in. I plan time to work so I can help my patients and clients improve their lives. You to have to plan time to create balance in your life. I love what I do and don't know if I will ever retire fully, but I am planning for time and money freedom so I can continue doing what I love and spending time with those that matter to me while making a difference in this world helping to improve the lives of others, who in turn, can make their own difference by making their dreams come true.

Chapter 12

Obstacles in Your Way

Take a deep breath and decide if you are ready to make the necessary changes to feel great and be super productive in everything you do. Know that you can do this, but you need to commit to doing what it takes. You need to look at your life now and then envision your life how you want it to be. When doing anything in life, either you're all in or you're all out. There is no maybe if you really want to see incredible results. However, I recommend you pick one or two steps that you can begin with right away, and then you can add a step every week so that you can implement the program easily and quickly. You may experience a resistance to change because what you're doing now is so familiar to you and even habitual. Sometimes it is hard to leave your comfort zone. However, if you want to reap the rewards of overcoming your fatigue, then I recommend you jump on board. The hardest part of this is deciding to do it and then taking the action steps needed. If you can decide to make the necessary changes to allow yourself to experience the full rewards, you will soon have greater energy and vitality and be super productive on and off the job. Be ready, willing, and able to make a change, and that will set you up for success. If you find that you are not getting it done, ask yourself if you truly want the result. If so, then take action and make the changes necessary to achieving success. Is your fatigue something you absolutely want to change? Yes or no? Maybe you think your problem isn't that bad because you're drinking so much caffeine to keep going? Listen to your heart and decide how you want to live your life. What does that life look like?

You might have even thought that your fatigue would go away on its own. I'm here to support you and lovingly remind you that if it were going to go away on its own, then it probably would have done so already. These are important choices for you to consider. Decide if it really is a problem you want to resolve. If so, do you want it to be just a little bit better, or are you wanting to change your life drastically? Before you can make a change, you have to decide.

Why wouldn't you want to resolve it? What do you gain by keeping it? Is now the right time for you to start this process? Are you too tired to change? Or maybe you think you can't do it on your own.

Look deeply into your soul and notice what you're feeling right now, and decide if you're longing for a better life. What is it costing you to say the same? What is it costing your family? What about your work? When you can see clearly all the pros and cons of making the changes necessary to taking all the steps to help yourself, then you will make the decision that is right for you. Do this for yourself and do it for the dream of a better life. A life you'd love to live.

What are other obstacles that could get in your way? Sometimes the lack of consistency in following the steps makes the process take longer or the results fall short of your dream. I want to encourage you to do what you can, and really add one or two steps a week or every other week until you are doing all eight of them. The steps can be added in any order and, while some people think drinking the water is the easiest step to add, if you are having trouble implementing the program, then may I suggest you start with mindset and the law of resonance. That way your thoughts will create certain feelings, and that will help you to take the actions necessary to get the results you want to see in your life.

Don't worry if you feel you may fail at doing all the steps. Worry is a waste of time and puts you in a downward spiral. Lift yourself up and think and feel that you have already achieved what you want. Remember the affirmation, "I am so happy and grateful now that _____." I am so happy and grateful now that I feel great and I am super productive at work. Let go of any fear or worry you may have, because it doesn't serve you. The main thing that is important is that you focus on what you want and take small action steps toward your goal. Ask yourself what you can do in the next seven days to move yourself in the direction of your goal. You can take little steps or big steps. I believe as long as the steps are done on a consistent basis with persistence to keep on doing them, then your life will be transformed.

When you have a win and you feel somewhat better, celebrate it and keep going until you achieve your dream come true. If you stop, you will only have a short-term success. If you want long-term success, keep going and see how you grow in energy and in health, wellness, and vitality. You will also grow as a person because you will have learned that in any success a winner never quits. Health is a lifestyle and, when you make the necessary changes in your life, you will see all the possibilities.

I knew a bodybuilder who was training for a competition and went through some incredible changes to have a winning physique and he won. He looked amazing and it was such hard work to get to that stage for him. He made many sacrifices to get there, and he was on cloud nine. On the way home from the competition, he stopped at a pizza place and ate two large pizzas. He went wild and, in a matter of days, you could see the added weight. In a matter of months, he just looked huge because he had all that muscle underneath a moderate amount of fat. The changes he made were drastic and unsustainable. I'm not advising you make crazy changes that are unsustainable or detrimental. I want to see a sustainable lifestyle change that benefits you for many years to come.

I have another client that works out four days a week and has done so for many years, and she eats a healthy plant-based diet and gets her adjustments and is a wonderful person in all the areas of her life. She looks and feels amazing. You couldn't get her to give that up because she wants to be happy and healthy for life, not just for a competition. In order to have the life you want, make the changes necessary and take the actions required. I have had a few clients that need to make changes in their lives, who are suffering and feel miserable. For them, I suggested they add different products and services that would help them achieve the best results and help them live the life they want to live. But they are in the research mode. They just gather information and gather more information and gather even more information and before you know it, they have all the information they need with no drive to take any action.

Let me stress to you that in order to make a positive change, you need to do something different than you are doing now. It only takes a minute to decide! Don't short change your success and progress by procrastinating.

Yes, research is a form of procrastination. If you truly want to get the results that are available to you, results that will change your life for the better, then you need to take action! I cannot stress it enough. If you have a dream it will never become a reality unless you take action steps in the direction of achieving it. I can tell you the people that get the best results in my clinic and through my coaching are the ones who take the action steps necessary to get from where they are to where they want to be. They are consistent with their treatment programs and persistent in everything they do. I heard a saying many years ago somewhere that stated, "how you do anything is how you do everything." I agree whole-heartedly. Decide to give it your all because this is your life and it will only be as good as you allow it to be. Decide and take action steps starting today.

Chapter 13

Conclusion

At the beginning of this book, you wanted to get your fatigue under control so that you didn't lose your job. You wanted to learn what to do so that you could feel great and be super productive in everything you do.

You learned that you are not alone and that fatigue is a modern epidemic, and there are steps you can do to increase your energy and productivity so that you can get your fatigue under control.

You learned that I have been through my own version of this myself, but more importantly, I have helped thousands of other people overcome their fatigue and become productive on and off the job.

You learned that you would have to decide to be open to change and do something differently so that you don't stay where you are, and you learned that there are eight exact steps to overcoming your fatigue so that you can feel great and be productive in everything you do.

You were able to understand how eating the right foods in the right proportions at the right times is critical to feeling great and being super energized and productive.

You were taught how drinking the right amount and type of water, and knowing when water should be consumed is critical to feeling great and being super productive at work.

You also learned about why it is so important for you to take vitamins, minerals, and redox signaling molecules to feel great and allow your body to function like it did when you were younger. You learned the difference between resting and sleeping, and the effect of sleep deprivation on your energy and what you need to do to get the right amount of sleep.

You also learned the effects of stress on the body physically, mentally, and biochemically, and how to minimize the effects of stress as much as possible. You learned how focused attitude and managing your emotions plays an important role in helping you feel great and be super productive at work, and you learned simple tips to benefiting from the law of resonance.

You learned that exercise, breathing, and stretching is imperative in helping you feel great and be super productive at work, and there are simple hacks you can do to fit it into your schedule.

You learned that mastering planning and time management will eliminate most of your mental stress.

And you learned that you will encounter some obstacles along the way in solving any problem, and that could jeopardize your success in feeling great and being super productive in everything you do. Being aware of those obstacles and having your focus on your action steps and doing them anyway will lead to success. All you have to do is decide to do it and then take the action steps needed.

My wish for you is that you will know you have all the tools you need to be truly successful at feeling great and being super productive in everything you do. Now, it's time to get it done. Most of the people I have worked with get it done. Some are able to accomplish it quickly and others may take a bit longer, but if you follow the steps and decide not to let anything get in your way, then you can have success, too. Don't be one of those people that collects information and doesn't implement what you have learned, otherwise you won't have the success you deserve.

Make a commitment to do something within five minutes of finishing this book. It doesn't have to be big, but it must be something that moves you in the right direction. Write down what you're going to start with and get started. Be committed, not just interested, in achieving the desired results. I believe the universe will give you absolutely anything you want as long as you're absolutely clear about what that is, so get clear. The time, money, energy, and effort spent investing in your health, heart, soul, and mind is time and energy and effort very well spent. You can't afford not to invest in yourself. Once there, keep investing every day, every week, every month, every year. Keep learning and keep growing and see where that takes you. Most of all, I hope you get to live the life you absolutely love.

Acknowledgements

When I was growing up my parents always supported their three daughters. They gave us the confidence and love to be able to pick our own path in life, and cheered us on with every accomplishment we had big or small. They were here for me through all the good times in my life and through adversity. I love you, Daddy, for always having my back and literally making me believe that I could do anything I put my mind to. There were a couple of times where the burden was great and I felt like quitting and you said, "keep going." I remember having a low point in my chiropractic school experience and I felt like I needed a change, and you said, "think of it as a prison sentence, stay the course, you're almost done and you can do it." It sounds funny now, but at the time you gave me the extra push I needed to keep going. Thank you for that and for always making yourself available to help me with anything I have ever needed. I know you love us all the same, but thank you for always making me feel like I am your favorite daughter. You and Mami shaped me into who I am today. Your love and support meant the world to me.

Thank you, Soren for putting up with me through this process and all the times I couldn't do things with you because I was working on this book and having to meet my deadlines. I'm so grateful for your love, support and encouragement. Thanks for always taking care of me in the process. I love you so much and appreciate you for giving me the space I needed when it was crunch time and for always making me take a break and bringing me lunch or dinner. I feel your love and I'm grateful for you every single day. I am so blessed to have you in my life.

Thank you Anisha for being such an amazing daughter and for inspiring me to be my best always, and thank you for forgiving me for some of those moments that I missed with you as a child. I love you! I'm so grateful for Braelin, Wesley, and Aurora and the love I feel when I think of you all. Your sweet little faces always gave me the extra lift I needed to push through the process and finish even when I was working into the wee hours of the morning.

Thank you, Dr. Miyoshi Feliciano, for being a wonderful sister and for all your words of encouragement while I was writing this book and, of course, throughout my life. Thank you for holding down the fort at the office when I had to work on this project and also when I wanted to see Ani and the grandkids. I am so grateful to have such a loving sister that I can always depend on to help me treat our wonderful patients when I am away as well as to help keep me healthy and aligned, too. Without your treatment after my accident, I wouldn't have been able to physically keep going and sit and write for the many hours it took for this project. I love you, sis!

Thank you Sahlly for being a wonderful big sister too, and for supporting me through this process and so much more, and all the free legal advice too. I love you sister, and I'm grateful for your willingness to always be there for me when I needed encouragement especially when I was so scared going through the medical tests. Thank you for dropping everything to hold my hand and support Soren as well.

I want to thank the rest of the family for all your love and encouragement too, and for cheering me on as I worked on this book and in everything I do. I love you all.

Thank you, Dr. Patti Giuliano for being my mentor and showing an unenthusiastic college student that I had so much more inside of me to bring to this world. You lit that spark inside of me to be a chiropractor and help enrich the lives of others, and I can't thank you enough for the wonderful life I have had since. There is no better feeling in the world than helping others. You were a wonderful example of who I wanted to become.

Thank you, Isabel Huizar for your support of me through this process and taking care of the clinic so that I didn't have to worry. I'm grateful that you share the same vision as I do in helping as many people as possible live happy and well. I hope you know that you are making an impact too.

I also want to thank all my practice consultants and coaches I have had over the years that helped me develop my programs and helped me manage my business, but I especially want to thank Dr. Gary Fieber for all the help you have given me personally in helping me change the lives of my clients. I appreciate the help and instruction you gave me especially as it relates to women's health and adrenal function testing. Thank you for helping both me and Isabel personally so that we were able to keep helping to change people's lives for the better.

I want to thank Dr. Dick Walker for always being accessible for me and my clients when I had any questions about redox signaling molecules and for also taking the time to clarify any questions that arose. You are a wealth of information and appreciate all your input and your willingness to help me and my clients out despite your busy schedule.

I want to thank all my patients and clients for your trust and confidence in me and for all your words of encouragement while I wrote this book. You all are so amazing and I'm so blessed and honored to be able to be part of your journey in health and vitality. You all mean the world to me and I am devoted to helping you live your best lives.

I also want to thank all my wonderful friends who kept calling me and texting me to see if I started writing and offered their love, support, and advice when they knew I was trying to make it all happen. Your words of support kept me going. Thank you all so very much!

The team at The Author Incubator has also asked me to acknowledge the Morgan James Publishing Team: David Hancock, CEO & Founder; my Author Relations Manager, Gayle West and special thanks to Jim Howard, Bethany Marshall, and Nickcole Watkins.

Thank You

Thank you for reading my book. This isn't the end but the beginning of a new journey. A journey that does not include fatigue. Imagine a life where you feel great and are super productive in everything you do! I find the most powerful way to begin is to get a complete picture of where you are now. This will help you know where to start and where to place your focus to get the best results. To get a complete picture of your energy level, what it'll take for you to feel great, and double or triple your productivity in everything you do, take my free energy quiz. Find out exactly where you are now and if working with me can make a difference for you. You will get the answers you need in less than five minutes. If you want to take the Energy Quiz, please go to **TheEnergyQuiz.com**.

Also there were extras that I wanted to include in this book that didn't make it in such as pictures, diagrams and additional information to make it easier to not only understand the material but to implement it that is compiled into a companion PDF. **Download the Free companion PDF to this book at NoMoreFatigueextras.com.**

About the Author

D r. Yani Feliciano is a chiropractor and health and wellness consultant who graduated from the Los Angeles College of Chiropractic in 1987. She has been in private practice in Whittier, California since

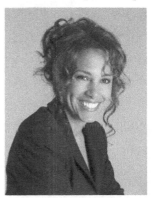

1987. She became a board qualified chiropractic orthopedist in 1990 after completing an extra 3 years of postgraduate study. As a qualified medical evaluator appointed by the State of California, she helps resolve disputes between injured workers and their employers.

Dr. Yani's mission is to "help as many people as possible live their lives to the fullest without pain or limitations!" She has been successful in achieving this by staying on top of cutting-edge technology in the health and wellness industry. When learning about new breakthroughs to help her clients, she researches them and tries them herself before recommending anything new to her clients. She is passionate about helping her clients overcome their limitations so that they can feel great and be super productive in everything they do. Dr. Yani uses a computer guided evaluation and treatment instrument that allows her to gently and precisely treat her patients without twisting, turning, or cracking the spine. It is extremely safe and the results are phenomenal.

Dr. Yani was voted Best Chiropractor in Whittier 2010 and 2011 and is featured on the "Best of LA" TV show regularly. Three years in a row, 2014-2016, she was awarded Best of the Best Chiropractor by the Whittier Area Chamber of Commerce. Dr. Yani devotes her time to patient care, one-on-one coaching, group coaching, and community education by presenting wellness workshops on a variety of topics including stress reduction and energy enhancements. Her workshops are filled with actionable steps that you can implement immediately to improve your health and eliminate your fatigue for good. She has been able to help thousands of people overcome their fatigue and improve their lives.

Dr. Yani is married and resides in Coto De Caza, California with her husband Soren and their Pomeranian, Teddy. In her spare time, Dr. Yani enjoys riding her beautiful Palomino, Joe, with her girlfriends, and boating up and down the California Riviera with her husband. She loves going up to Washington State to visit her daughter, son in law, and her three beautiful grandchildren as often as possible. She has been known to humor her grandkids while accompanying them down the Great Wolf Lodge water park slides.

She is involved in several groups and organizations, but her passion and heart belongs to Soroptimist International of Whittier, an organization that helps women and girls in her local community and throughout the world. A portion of the proceeds from this book will be donated to them.

To contact Dr. Yani for any speaking engagements or workshop opportunities please email her at docyani46@gmail.com

Website: proadjusterchiropractic.net
Email: docyani46@gmail.com
Facebook: Yani Feliciano
Facebook: Friends Chiropractic
LinkedIn: Yani Feliciano